VASCULAR RESEARCH DEVELOPMENTS

THE VSITE REVIEW

VASCULAR RESEARCH DEVELOPMENTS

Additional books and e-books in this series can be found on Nova's website under the Series tab.

VASCULAR RESEARCH DEVELOPMENTS

THE VSITE REVIEW

YOUNG KIM

nova science publishers
New York

NOTICE TO THE READER

The Publisher has taken reasonable care in the preparation of this book, but makes no expressed or implied warranty of any kind and assumes no responsibility for any errors or omissions. No liability is assumed for incidental or consequential damages in connection with or arising out of information contained in this book. The Publisher shall not be liable for any special, consequential, or exemplary damages resulting, in whole or in part, from the readers' use of, or reliance upon, this material. Any parts of this book based on government reports are so indicated and copyright is claimed for those parts to the extent applicable to compilations of such works.

Independent verification should be sought for any data, advice or recommendations contained in this book. In addition, no responsibility is assumed by the Publisher for any injury and/or damage to persons or property arising from any methods, products, instructions, ideas or otherwise contained in this publication.

This publication is designed to provide accurate and authoritative information with regard to the subject matter covered herein. It is sold with the clear understanding that the Publisher is not engaged in rendering legal or any other professional services. If legal or any other expert assistance is required, the services of a competent person should be sought. FROM A DECLARATION OF PARTICIPANTS JOINTLY ADOPTED BY A COMMITTEE OF THE AMERICAN BAR ASSOCIATION AND A COMMITTEE OF PUBLISHERS.

Additional color graphics may be available in the e-book version of this book.

Library of Congress Cataloging-in-Publication Data

Names: Kim, Young (MD), author.
Title: The VSITE review / Young Kim.
Description: New York : Nova Science Publishers, [2021] | Series: Vascular research developments | Includes bibliographical references and index. |
Identifiers: LCCN 2021038503 (print) | LCCN 2021038504 (ebook) | ISBN 9781536199345 (hardcover) | ISBN 9781685070304 (adobe pdf)
Subjects: LCSH: Blood-vessels--Surgery--Outlines, syllabi, etc.
Classification: LCC RD598.5 K56 2021 (print) | LCC RD598.5 (ebook) | DDC 617.4/13--dc23
LC record available at https://lccn.loc.gov/2021038503
LC ebook record available at https://lccn.loc.gov/2021038504

Published by Nova Science Publishers, Inc. † New York

CONTENTS

PREFACE

Each disease process has been broken down into an outline format, emphasizing etiology, clinical presentation, classification schemes, relevant risk factors, and current principles in management. Management is further divided into diagnostic tests and treatment options, including any surgical procedures and indications for surgery. This book is strictly for review purposes, and is not designed to be used as a guideline in clinical decision making.

Chapter 1

Cerebrovascular Review

Overview

- Carotid Artery Stenosis
- Carotid Artery Occlusion
- Carotid Artery Restenosis
- Carotid Artery Fibromuscular Dysplasia (FMD)
- Concomitant Carotid/Coronary Artery Stenosis
- Carotid Artery Kinks/Coils
- Carotid Artery Aneurysm
- Carotid Body Tumor
- Vertebral Artery Stenosis
- Subclavian Artery Stenosis
- Innominate Artery Stenosis
- Giant Cell Arteritis (Temporal Arteritis)
- Takayasu Arteritis
- Radiation Arteritis
- Stroke (Post-CEA)
- Cranial Nerve Injury (Post-CEA)

- Cerebral Hyperperfusion Syndrome
- Infected Carotid Patch

Carotid Artery Stenosis

- Etiology
    - Atherosclerotic plaque forms at carotid bifurcation due to hemodynamic conditions
    - Plaques become clinically significant due to stenosis, occlusion, or embolization
- Presentation
    - Asymptomatic
    - Neurologic deficits
        - Contralateral sensorimotor deficits, aphasia/dysphasia, ipsilateral amaurosis fugax
        - Amaurosis fugax: retinal artery atheroembolic plaque causes monocular visual deficit
        - Transient ischemic attack (TIA): focal neurologic deficit that lasts <24 hrs
            - Crescendo TIA: repeat deficits with complete return to baseline between attacks
        - Reversible ischemic neurologic deficit (RIND): focal neurologic deficit that lasts 24-48 hrs
        - Stroke (CVA): focal neurologic deficit that lasts >48 hrs
            - Stroke-in-evolution: clinically worsening deficits without return to normal baseline
- Risk factors
    - Atherosclerosis (hypertension, hyperlipidemia, smoking, diabetes, male gender)
- Management
    - Diagnosis

        - Carotid duplex
            - <50% stenosis: PSV <125 cm/sec, I:C PSV ratio <2, EDV <40
            - 50-69% stenosis: PSV 125-230 cm/sec, I:C PSV ratio 2-4, EDV 40-100
            - 70-99% stenosis: PSV >230 cm/sec, I:C PSV ratio >4, EDV >100
        - CT/MR angiogram
        - Conventional angiogram
            - "Gold standard" but invasive, risk of stroke
- Treatment
    - Medical management
        - Aspirin, smoking cessation, exercise, healthy diet
        - Treat hypertension (<140/90), diabetes (A1c <7%), hyperlipidemia (LDL <100 or <70 for diabetics)
        - Surgical options
            - Carotid endarterectomy
                - ✓ Two methods - endarterectomy/patch angioplasty, eversion endarterectomy
                - ✓ Eversion indicated for carotid kinks/coils
                - ✓ Techniques to reach high bifurcation - nasotracheal intubation, divide posterior belly of digastric, anterior mandibular subluxation, divide styloid process
            - Carotid artery stenting (transfemoral)
                - ✓ Reserved for high-risk symptomatic patients only
            - Trans-carotid artery revascularization (TCAR)
                - ✓ Reserved for high-risk symptomatic patients only

- ✓ Requires 5 cm length between proximal CCA and bifurcation

- ▪ Indications for surgery
  - – Severe symptomatic stenosis (70-99%)
  - – Risk-benefit analysis for moderate symptomatic stenosis (50-69% in men)
  - – Severe asymptomatic stenosis (60-99%)
  - – Optimal timing is 2-14 days after onset of symptoms
  - – *Emergent* CEA for stroke-in-evolution or crescendo TIA
  - – Life expectancy <2 years is a contraindication to surgery
- ▪ Follow-up
  - – Carotid duplex
    - ✓ Timing - 30 days, 6/12/18/24 mo, annual afterwards

- Studies
  - o NASCET trial: CEA has reduced stroke in symptomatic stenosis >70% (26% vs 9%, 2 yrs)
  - o ECST trial: CEA has reduced stroke in symptomatic stenosis >80% (16.8% vs 2.8%, 3 yrs)
  - o ACAS trial: CEA has reduced stroke in asymptomatic stenosis >60% (11% vs 5.1%, 5 yrs)
  - o CREST trial: CEA has higher MI (2.3% vs 1.1%), CAS has higher stroke (4.1% vs 2.3%)

Carotid Artery Occlusion

- Etiology
  - Complete occlusion (100% stenosis) of ICA
  - Carotid stump syndrome: turbulent flow in occluded ICA stump promotes atheroembolization through ECA collaterals
- Presentation
  - Asymptomatic
  - Neurologic deficits
- Management
  - Diagnosis
    - Carotid duplex
    - CT/MR angiogram
      - Make sure to check delayed phase
  - Treatment
    - Medical management
      - Aspirin, smoking cessation, exercise, healthy diet
      - Treat hypertension (<140/90), diabetes (A1c <7%), hyperlipidemia (LDL <100 or <70 for diabetics)
    - Surgical options
      - ECA endarterectomy with ICA stumpectomy
        - ✓ Ligate ICA flush with CCA
        - ✓ Postoperative anticoagulation
      - Extracranial-intracranial (EC-IC) bypass
        - ✓ Bypass from ECA branch (STA) to MCA using radial artery
        - ✓ No benefit over medical management
    - Indications for surgery
      - Symptomatic occlusion

CAROTID ARTERY RESTENOSIS

- Etiology
  - >50% reduction in carotid diameter after CEA or CAS
  - Multiple etiologies depending on time course
    - Technical error if within 30 days
    - Neointimal hyperplasia if 30 days – 2 yrs
    - Recurrent atherosclerosis if after 2 yrs
  - Rate of restenosis is 10% (first year), 3% (second year), 1% (annually afterwards)
- Presentation
  - Asymptomatic finding on follow-up duplex
  - Neurologic deficits
- Risk factors
  - Female gender, primary closure without patch angioplasty, smoking
- Management
  - Diagnosis
    - Carotid duplex
      - 50% stenosis: PSV >220 cm/sec
      - 80% stenosis: PSV >340 cm/sec
    - CT/MR angiogram
  - Treatment
    - Medical management
      - Aspirin, smoking cessation, exercise, healthy diet
      - Treat hypertension (<140/90), diabetes (A1c <7%), hyperlipidemia (LDL <100 or <70 for diabetes)
    - Surgical options
      - Repeat carotid endarterectomy
      - Carotid resection with interposition graft
      - Carotid-subclavian bypass
      - Carotid-carotid bypass

- Carotid artery stenting (transfemoral)
  - ✓ No long-term comparison results between CEA vs CAS
- Indications for surgery
  - Symptomatic restenosis (>50%)
  - Asymptomatic restenosis (>80%)

CAROTID ARTERY FIBROMUSCULAR DYSPLASIA (FMD)

- Etiology
  - Stenotic segments due to medial fibrodysplasia (most common type)
    - Replacement of media by disorganized myofibroblasts
    - Aneurysmal dilations form between stenotic segments due to thinning of media
  - Clinically relevant with flow reduction, thrombus formation, embolization, dissection
  - 65% have bilateral disease
- Presentation
  - Asymptomatic
  - Neurologic deficits
- Risk factors
  - Female gender (85%)
- Management
  - Diagnosis
    - Carotid duplex
    - CT/MR angiogram
    - "String-of-beads" appearance
    - Rule-out intracranial aneurysms (13% incidence)
  - Treatment
    - Medical management

        - Aspirin (for asymptomatic disease)
    - Surgical options
        - Graduated intraluminal dilation (for stenosis)
        - Resection with interposition graft (for aneurysms)
        - Carotid artery angioplasty
            - ✓ Rescue stenting indicated only for flow-limiting dissection or thrombus-containing pseudo-aneurysms
    - Indications for surgery
        - Symptomatic lesions

Concomitant Carotid/Coronary Artery Stenosis

- Etiology
  - Coexistent carotid and coronary artery disease
- Presentation
  - Carotid artery disease can be symptomatic (neurological deficits) or asymptomatic
  - Coronary artery disease can be stable (angina) or unstable (acute infarction)
- Management
  - Diagnosis
    - Carotid evaluation
      - Carotid duplex
      - CT/MR angiogram
    - Coronary evaluation
      - Echocardiogram
      - Left heart catheterization
      - Stress test
  - Treatment
    - Staged procedure (CEA then CABG)

    - Ideal for symptomatic or severe bilateral carotid stenosis
  - Reversed-staged procedure (CABG then CEA)
  - Concomitant procedure (combined CEA/CABG)
    - No consensus regarding optimal treatment approach

Carotid Artery Dissection

- Etiology
  - Two mechanisms of injury
    - Stretch-traction-rotation injury
    - Compression injury between mandible and cervical vertebrae
  - Can result from trauma, violent coughing, emesis, heavy exercise, chiropractic manipulation
- Presentation
  - Asymptomatic finding during trauma evaluation
  - Neurologic symptoms, severe hemicrania ("throbbing" ipsilateral head/neck pain), Horner syndrome
- Risk factors
  - Carotid FMD, kinks/coils, temporal arteritis, collagen vascular disorders
- Management
  - Diagnosis
    - Carotid duplex
    - Conventional angiogram
    - CT/MR angiogram
      - Tapered narrowing of distal bulb/proximal ICA
  - Treatment
    - Medical management
      - Antiplatelets vs anticoagulation

        - ✓ No good comparison studies
      - – Repeat CTA prior to discharge
    - Surgical options
      - – Open carotid repair
      - – Carotid artery stenting
    - Indications for surgery
      - – Failure of medical management (worsening neurologic deficits), flow-limiting lesions, symptomatic or enlarging pseudoaneurysm

CAROTID ARTERY KINKS/COILS

- Etiology
  - Coil: vessel elongation in confined space results in coiling
  - Kink: vessel degeneration results in acute angulation <90°
- Presentation
  - Asymptomatic
  - Neurologic deficits
- Classification (Togay-Isikay criteria)
  - Mild kink (grade I): 60-90° angulation
  - Moderate kink (grade II): 30-60° angulation
  - Severe kink (grade III): <30° angulation
  - Tortuosity: S- or C-shaped course of ICA
  - Coil: exaggerated S-shape or circular configuration of ICA
- Management
  - Diagnosis
    - Carotid duplex
      - – Lack of post-stenotic turbulence can help differentiate kink/coil from atherosclerotic stenosis
    - CT/MR angiogram
  - Treatment

- Surgical options
  - Division and reimplantation of ICA into proximal CCA
  - Excision of redundant ICA and reimplantation into CCA
  - Excision of redundant ICA with bypass grafting
  - Mobilization and resection of CCA with CCA-CCA anastomosis
  - Transposition of ICA onto ECA
- Indications for surgery
  - Symptomatic kinks/coils

CAROTID ARTERY ANEURYSM

- Etiology
  - True carotid aneurysms
    - Carotid artery diameter >1.5 cm
    - Majority (>95%) located at carotid bulb
  - False carotid aneurysms
    - Secondary to trauma or post-endarterectomy
- Presentation
  - Pulsatile neck mass with *negative* Fontaine sign
  - Neurologic deficits (thromboembolism), mass effect (cranial nerve compression), or rupture (rare)
- Management
  - Diagnosis
    - Carotid duplex
    - CT/MR angiogram
  - Treatment
    - Surgical options
      - Carotid artery covered stenting

- Aneurysmectomy with local reconstruction
- Aneurysmectomy with carotid-carotid interposition graft

▪ Indications for surgery
  - All aneurysms and pseudoaneurysms

CAROTID BODY TUMOR

- Etiology
  - Cervical paraganglioma located within the adventitial layer of common carotid bifurcation
    - 75% sporadic, 25% associated with family history
  - Rarely (5%) metastasizes to lymph nodes, liver, lung, bone, brain
  - Meyer ligament: blood supply from ECA feeder vessels, most commonly ascending pharyngeal artery
- Presentation
  - Pulsatile neck mass with *positive* Fontaine sign
  - Mass effect (cranial nerve compression)
  - Fontaine sign: lateral displacement of neck mass results in movement of carotid pulse in same direction
- Classification (Shamblin)
  - Group I tumors: abut ICA/ECA
  - Group II tumors: partially encase ICA/ECA
  - Group III tumors: completely encase ICA/ECA
- Risk factors
  - *SDH* mutation predisposes to familial tumors (often bilateral)
  - Higher altitudes cause chronic hypoxia and carotid body cell hyperplasia
- Management

- Diagnosis
  - Carotid duplex
  - CT/MR angiogram
    - Lyre sign: hypervascular mass splaying bifurcation
  - Genetic testing
    - Indicated for positive family history, multifocal tumors, history of previous pheochromocytoma/ paraganglioma
- Treatment
  - Surgical options
    - Preoperative embolization
      - ✓ Indicated for Shamblin II/III tumors
      - ✓ Selective for ascending pharyngeal branch
      - ✓ Should precede resection by 24-36 hrs
    - Carotid body tumor resection
      - ✓ Dissect along periadventitial plane
      - ✓ 5% cranial nerve injury, 1-2% stroke risk

VERTEBRAL ARTERY STENOSIS

- Etiology
  - Vertebral artery stenosis or occlusion results in decreased blood flow to brainstem/cerebellum
  - Low flow state precipitated by hypotension
  - Usually compensated via collateral flow through Circle of Willis
- Presentation
  - Asymptomatic
  - Vertebrobasilar insufficiency (VBI)
    - Dizziness, vertigo, diplopia, blurry vision, tinnitus, drop attacks

  - Bow hunter syndrome: head rotation causes compression of V3 segment resulting in VBI symptoms
- Anatomy
  - V1 segment: preforaminal, subclavian artery to C6 transverse foramen
  - V2 segment: foraminal, C6 to C2 transverse foramina
  - V3 segment: extradural, C2 transverse foramen to dura mater
  - V4 segment: intradural, dura mater to basilar artery
    - Only V1 and V3 segments are surgically accessible
- Management
  - Diagnosis
    - CT/MR angiogram (gold standard)
    - Conventional angiogram
    - Dynamic angiogram
      - Indicated for rotational symptoms
  - Treatment
    - Medical management
      - Aspirin, smoking cessation, exercise, healthy diet
      - Treat hypertension (<140/90), diabetes (A1c <7%), hyperlipidemia (LDL <100 or <70 for diabetics)
    - Surgical options
      - Carotid-vertebral transposition (V1 stenosis)
        - ✓ 20% risk of Horner syndrome
      - Carotid-distal vertebral bypass (V1 or V2 stenosis)
      - C1 posterior laminectomy
        - ✓ Indicated for bow hunter syndrome
    - Indications for surgery
      - Symptomatic stenosis (dominant side only)

Subclavian Artery Stenosis

- Etiology
  - Subclavian artery stenosis results in SBP difference >15 mmHg
- Presentation
  - Asymptomatic (>90%)
  - Ipsilateral exertional arm ischemia (limb fatigue, pain, heaviness)
    - More likely to have symptoms with SBP gradient >40 mmHg
  - Subclavian steal syndrome: proximal subclavian artery stenosis decreases perfusion to distal subclavian artery and ipsilateral vertebral artery, resulting in reversal of vertebral artery flow and VBI symptoms with arm exercise
- Anatomy
  - First segment: medial to anterior scalene
    - Internal mammary artery, vertebral artery, thyrocervical trunk
  - Second segment: deep to anterior scalene
    - Superior intercostal artery, deep cervical artery
  - Third segment: lateral to anterior scalene
    - Dorsal scapular artery
    - Becomes axillary artery at lateral border of 1st rib
- Management
  - Diagnosis
    - Duplex ultrasound
      - Bidirectional or retrograde vertebral flow
      - CT/MR angiogram
      - Conventional angiogram
  - Treatment
    - Medical management

        - Aspirin, smoking cessation, exercise, healthy diet
        - Treat hypertension (<140/90), diabetes (A1c <7%), hyperlipidemia (LDL <100 or <70 for diabetics)
    - Surgical options
        - Carotid-subclavian transposition
        - Carotid-subclavian bypass
            - ✓ Long-term patency rates 10-15% lower than transposition
        - Axillo-axillary bypass
            - ✓ Indicated for hostile neck
        - Subclavian angioplasty/stenting
            - ✓ Contraindicated with ostial occlusion, coverage of vertebral arteries
        - Indications for surgery
            - ✓ Symptomatic stenosis, severe bilateral disease (for BP monitoring), pre-CABG (LIMA conduit), or pre-TEVAR (extend proximal landing zone)

INNOMINATE ARTERY STENOSIS

- Etiology
    - Innominate artery stenosis results in decreased perfusion to right brain and right upper extremity
    - Presentation
    - Asymptomatic
    - Subclavian symptoms – right exertional arm ischemia (limb fatigue, pain, heaviness)
    - Carotid symptoms – neurologic deficits
    - Vertebral symptoms – vertebrobasilar insufficiency
- Management
    - Diagnosis

        - Duplex ultrasound
        - CT/MR angiogram
        - Conventional angiogram
    - Treatment
        - Medical management
            - Aspirin, smoking cessation, exercise, healthy diet
            - Treat hypertension (<140/90), diabetes (A1c <7%), hyperlipidemia (LDL <100 or <70 for diabetics)
        - Surgical options
            - Aorto-innominate bypass (gold standard)
                - ✓ Contraindicated with heavy calcification or extensive intraluminal thrombus
            - Innominate endarterectomy
                - ✓ Ideal for focal lesions
            - Carotid-carotid-subclavian bypass
                - ✓ Ideal for high-risk patients or hostile chest
                - ✓ Retropharyngeal tunnel with 8 mm ringed PTFE graft
            - Innominate angioplasty/stenting
                - ✓ Ideal for focal lesions
                - ✓ Long-term patency rates unknown
        - Indications for surgery
            - Symptomatic stenosis (>50%), asymptomatic stenosis (>80%)

GIANT CELL ARTERITIS (TEMPORAL ARTERITIS)

- Etiology
    - Inflammatory arteritis of medium and large vessels
    - Involves aorta, carotid arteries, temporal arteries
- Presentation

- Temporal headache with scalp tenderness, jaw claudication
- Monocular vision loss due to ischemic optic neuropathy from ciliary artery involvement

- Risk factors
  - Female gender, old age, polymyalgia rheumatica
- Management
  - Diagnosis
  - American College of Rheumatology criteria (need 3 of 5)
    - Age >50
    - ESR >50
    - New-onset headache
    - Temporal artery abnormality (tenderness or decreased pulse)
    - Abnormal biopsy result
  - CT/MR angiogram
  - Temporal artery biopsy (>2 cm)
    - Transmural inflammation with multinucleated giant cells
    - 42% false negative rate
  - Treatment
  - Medical management
    - Corticosteroids
    - Tocilizumab (IL-6 antibody)

TAKAYASU ARTERITIS

- Etiology
  - Inflammatory arteritis of medium and large vessels
  - Involves aorta and proximal branches
- Presentation
  - Acute systemic phase

        - Active inflammatory illness with constitutional symptoms (fever, fatigue, weight loss), arterial tenderness
        - Carotidynia is pathognomonic finding for Takayasu arteritis
    - Chronic occlusive phase
        - Segmental stenoses and aneurysms with end-organ ischemia
        - Symptoms vary with involved vessels
            - Renal symptoms – renovascular hypertension (most common)
            - Subclavian symptoms – extremity ischemia
            - Carotid symptoms – neurologic symptoms
- Classification (Tokyo International Conference Classifi-cation)
    - Type I: arch vessels
    - Type IIa: arch vessels, ascending aorta
    - Type IIb: arch vessels, ascending aorta, thoracic descending aorta
    - Type III: thoracic descending aorta, abdominal aorta, renal arteries
    - Type IV: abdominal aorta, renal arteries
    - Type V: all of the above (most common type)
- Risk factors
    - Female gender (>80%), Asian ethnicity
- Management
    - Diagnosis
        - CT/MR angiogram (gold standard)
        - "Skip lesions"
        - Conventional angiogram
    - Treatment
        - Medical management
            - Corticosteroids

- Indicated for systemic phase
- High relapse rates
- Surgical options
  - Open bypass
    - ✓ Resection with interposition graft
  - Proximal and distal anastomosis should be free of inflammation
  - Angioplasty
    - ✓ High rate of restenosis, short-term relief only
- Indications for surgery
  - Occlusive phase with symptomatic stenoses

Radiation Arteritis

- Etiology
  - Segmental arteritis secondary to radiation injury
  - Arterial involvement varies with field of radiation treatment
    - Subclavian-axillary injury due to breast radiation
    - Aortic, visceral, renal injury due to abdominal radiation
    - External iliac injury due to uterine/prostate radiation
    - SFA injury due to sarcoma radiation
  - Venous involvement is extremely rare
- Presentation
  - Carotid lesions – neurologic deficits
  - Subclavian-axillary lesions – ipsilateral exertional arm ischemia
  - Renal lesions – renovascular hypertension
  - Aortoiliac lesions – lower extremity ischemia
- Risk factors
  - Atherosclerosis (hypertension, hyperlipidemia, smoking, diabetes, male gender)

- Management
  - Diagnosis
    - CT/MR angiogram
      - Smooth, tapered lesions in atypical locations
    - Conventional angiogram
  - Treatment
    - Surgical options (varies by location)
      - Endarterectomy
      - Resection with interposition graft
      - Bypass graft without resection
      - Angioplasty/stenting
        - ✓ Ideal for focal lesions
    - Indications for surgery
      - Symptomatic stenoses

STROKE (POST-CEA)

- Etiology
  - Hypoperfusion during carotid clamping
  - Thrombosis or embolization from endarterectomy site
- Presentation
  - Neurologic deficits recognized after carotid endarterectomy
- Risk factors
  - Intraoperative hypotension
- Management
  - Diagnosis
    - Intraoperative diagnosis
      - Regional anesthesia
      - EEG monitoring
        - ✓ >50% reduction in waveform amplitude
      - Stump pressures

      - ✓ <40 mmHg
    - Postoperative diagnosis
      - Duplex ultrasound
      - CT angiogram
  - Treatment
    - If hypoperfusion →
      - Carotid shunting
      - Vasopressor support
    - If thrombus →
      - Thrombectomy
    - If embolization →
      - Catheter-directed TPA
      - Mechanical thrombectomy

Cranial Nerve Injury (Post-CEA)

- Etiology
  - Technical error or retraction injury during carotid endarterectomy
- Presentation
  - Marginal mandibular injury: ipsilateral lip droop
  - Hypoglossal injury: ipsilateral tongue deviation
  - Glossopharyngeal injury: dysphagia, aspiration risk
  - Vagus injury: hoarseness
- Risk factors
  - Neck radiation, reoperative field
- Management
  - Diagnosis
    - Neurologic exam
  - Treatment
    - Supportive care

CEREBRAL HYPERPERFUSION SYNDROME

- Etiology
  - Chronic severe carotid occlusive disease results in fixed maximal vasodilation
  - Removal of obstructive plaque causes increased cerebral blood flow due to loss of autoregulation
  - Hyperperfusion can cause cerebral edema and vessel rupture if severe
- Presentation
  - Hypertension, ipsilateral headache, can progress to seizures and hemorrhagic stroke
  - Median onset of symptoms between POD#3-5
- Risk factors
  - Postoperative hypertension, preoperative stroke, high-grade carotid stenosis (>90%), anticoagulation, chronic cerebral ischemia
- Management
  - Diagnosis
    - CT head
      - Rule-out stroke
    - EEG
      - Periodic lateralizing epileptiform discharges
  - Treatment
    - Medical management
      - Control hypertension (SBP<140)
      - Diuretics (decrease swelling), steroids
      - Consider neurosurgery consult
  - Prevention
    - Blood pressure control (SBP <140)

INFECTED CAROTID PATCH

- Etiology
  - *Staphylococcus* (>90%), *Streptococcus, Bacteroides, Pseudomonas, Proteus* spp.
- Presentation
  - Abscess, complex wound infection, patch rupture, false aneurysm, chronic sinus discharge
  - Bimodal distribution – majority present within 2 months or after 6 months
- Management
  - Diagnosis
    - Carotid duplex
    - CT/MR angiogram
  - Treatment
    - Medical management
      - IV antibiotics (no consensus on duration)
      - Tissue cultures
    - Surgical options
      - Patch excision with autologous tissue reconstruction

Chapter 2

UPPER EXTREMITY REVIEW

OVERVIEW

- Upper Extremity Occlusive Disease
- Raynaud Syndrome
- Buerger Disease (Thromboangiitis Obliterans)
- Ergotism (Ergotoxicosis)
- Neurogenic Thoracic Outlet Syndrome (NTOS)
- Venous Thoracic Outlet Syndrome (VTOS)
- Arterial Thoracic Outlet Syndrome (ATOS)
- Pectoralis Minor Syndrome
- Aberrant Right Subclavian Artery (Arteria Lusoria)
- Subclavian Artery Aneurysm
- Axillary Artery Aneurysm
- Hypothenar Hammer Syndrome (HHS)

UPPER EXTREMITY OCCLUSIVE DISEASE

- Etiology
  - Vasospasm
    - Most common cause of UE ischemia
    - Raynaud syndrome, ergotism, pressors, cocaine use
  - Intrinsic arterial disease
    - Atherosclerosis (<5%)
    - Azotemic arteriopathy
    - Radiation arteritis
    - Inflammatory arteritis
    - Takayasu arteritis
    - Giant cell arteritis
    - Buerger disease
  - Embolism
    - Cardiac source
    - Atheroembolism
    - Arterial TOS
  - Trauma
    - Blunt/penetrating trauma
    - Iatrogenic trauma (A-lines)
    - Occupational trauma
- Presentation
  - Asymptomatic
  - Symptomatic
    - Exercise-induced fatigue, Raynaud phenomenon, pain, claudication
    - Digital ischemia (cold fingers/toes, ischemic ulcerations, petechiae, splinter hemorrhage)
- Management
  - Diagnosis
    - Duplex ultrasound

        - CT/MR angiogram
        - Conventional angiogram
        - Gold standard
        - Significant variability in arterial anatomy
    - Treatment
        - Surgical options
            - Open bypass with vein graft
            - Open thrombectomy/endarterectomy with vein patch
            - Open embolectomy (embolic)
            - Angioplasty
                - ✓ No evidence for endovascular approach in chronic UE ischemia
            - Catheter-directed TPA

RAYNAUD SYNDROME

- Etiology
    - Primary Raynaud syndrome: primary vasospastic disease, diagnosis of exclusion
    - Secondary Raynaud syndrome: secondary to connective tissue disorders, medications, or other inciting factors
        - Ergotamine, vasopressors, cocaine, beta-blockers
- Presentation
    - Fingers/toes become white (pallor), then blue (cyanosis), then red (hyperemia)
    - Tissue loss only seen with secondary Raynaud syndrome
- Risk factors
    - Female gender (80%), young age (10-30 yo)
- Management
    - Diagnosis

        - Clinical diagnosis
            - Rule-out alternative diagnoses
            - Consider hypercoagulable work-up
            - Consider serologic screening
        - Nailfold capillary microscopy
            - Distorted capillary loops, capillary loss
        - Conventional angiogram
            - Indicated for tissue loss
    - Treatment
        - Medical management
            - Hand warmers, avoid triggers
            - Nifedipine, losartan
            - Treat underlying cause (if secondary)
        - Surgical options
            - Sympathectomy
                - ✓ Short-term relief
                - ✓ Ideal for toe symptoms, less durable for fingers

BUERGER DISEASE (THROMBOANGIITIS OBLITERANS)

- Etiology
    - Non-atherosclerotic inflammatory disease of medium/small vessels of extremities
    - Exact etiology is unknown but likely related to endothelial cell dysfunction
- Presentation
    - Digital ischemia (cold fingers/toes, ischemic ulcerations, petechiae, splinter hemorrhage)
- Risk factors
    - Smoking, male gender, young age
- Management

- Diagnosis
  - Shionoya criteria (need 4/5)
    - Smoking history (current or recent)
    - Age <50 yo
    - Infrapopliteal arterial occlusions
    - Upper extremity involvement or migratory thrombophlebitis
    - Absence of atherosclerotic risk factors
  - Duplex ultrasound
  - Conventional angiogram
    - Corkscrew collaterals
- Treatment
  - Medical management
    - Smoking cessation
      - ✓ Only intervention to stop disease progression
    - Intramuscular VEGF injections
    - Local wound care
  - Surgical options
    - T2/T3 sympathectomy (short-term relief)
    - Amputation (last line)

ERGOTISM (ERGOTOXICOSIS)

- Etiology
  - Ergot alkaloids act as agonists on serotonin, dopamine, α-adrenergic receptors
    - Causes powerful vasoconstriction
    - Clinically used to treat migraine and cluster headaches
  - Can be found in fungus-contaminated rye bread
  - Long-term ergot use results in prolonged vasoconstrictive activity

- Presentation
  - Two different sets of symptoms
  - Convulsive ergotism
    - Gastrointestinal symptoms include nausea, vomiting, diarrhea
    - Neurologic symptoms include headaches, tonic-clonic spasms, seizures, hallucinations, delirium
    - Usually GI symptoms precede CNS effects
  - Gangrenous ergotism (St. Anthony's fire)
    - Mild limb pain followed by "burning" shooting pain
    - Proceeds to loss of sensation, pulselessness, tissue loss, and autoamputation
- Risk factors
  - Smoking, chronic high-dose ergotamine use, cytochrome P450 inhibition
- Management
  - Diagnosis
    - Clinical diagnosis
    - Conventional angiogram
  - Treatment
    - Medical management
    - Smoking cessation, discontinue ergot-containing medications
    - Vasodilators (nifedipine, prazosin, nitroprusside)

Neurogenic Thoracic Outlet Syndrome (NTOS)

- Etiology
  - Brachial plexus compression within scalene triangle
    - Anterior scalene hypertrophy, injury, or fibrosis results in narrowing of thoracic outlet

        - Compression results in local pain and inflammation of brachial plexus, leading to edema and further narrowing of scalene triangle space
    - 95% of TOS
- Presentation
    - Upper extremity pain, parasthesias, weakness, numbness
    - Occipital headache secondary to upper trapezius/paraspinal muscle spasms
    - Hypothenar/thenar muscle atrophy (Gilliat-Sumner hand)
- Anatomy
    - Subclavius muscle/tendon lies underneath clavicle
    - Anterior scalene connects C3-C6 TP to scalene tubercle in 1st rib
        - Subclavian vein lies anterior to anterior scalene
        - Phrenic nerve courses laterally along anterior scalene, then behind subclavian vein
    - Middle scalene connects C2-C7 TP to scalene tubercle in 1st rib
        - Subclavian artery lies anterior to middle scalene
        - Brachial plexus (trunks) lies anterior to middle scalene
        - Long thoracic nerve courses through middle scalene
- Risk factors
    - Cervical rib or abnormal first rib
    - Poor posture, neck trauma, whiplash injury, work-related injury, overuse activities, previous clavicle fracture
- Management
    - Diagnosis
        - Physical exam (gold standard)
            - Scalene triangle tenderness, exacerbation of symptoms with palpation
            - Upper limb tension test (ULTT): extend arms at 90 degrees and flex/extend wrists repeatedly

- Elevated arm stress test (EAST): open and close hands in "surrender" position for three minutes
- Chest X-ray
  - ✓ Cervical rib or abnormal first rib (not always present)
- CT/MRI chest/neck
  - ✓ Rule-out alternative diagnoses
- EMG/nerve conduction study (unreliable)

- Treatment
  - Medical management
    - Physical therapy
      - ✓ First-line due to high recurrence rate with surgical decompression
      - ✓ 80-90% successful with prolonged physical therapy
    - Modification of work environment to prevent postural imbalances
    - Scalene muscle block
      - ✓ Offered after 3-6 months of physical therapy if no response
      - ✓ Helps determine which patients are likely to have symptomatic relief after surgery
- Surgical options
  - Thoracic outlet decompression
    - First rib resection, anterior scalenectomy
    - Transaxillary approach
      - ✓ Advantages - cosmetically appealing, ideal for small ribs
      - ✓ Disadvantages - inability to perform large rib resection or vascular repair, can't manipulate shoulder if prior shoulder surgery
      - ✓ Supraclavicular approach

    - ✓ Advantages - ideal for arterial reconstruction, larger ribs
  - – Infraclavicular approach
    - ✓ Advantages - ideal for venous reconstruction, pec minor release

VENOUS THORACIC OUTLET SYNDROME (VTOS, PAGET-SCHROETTER SYNDROME)

- Etiology
  - Subclavian vein compression between clavicle and cervical rib
    - Extrinsic compression results in intimal hyperplasia and venous thrombosis
  - 4% of TOS
- Presentation
  - Acute-onset upper extremity pain, edema (non-pitting), cyanosis
  - Prominent collateral veins over shoulder, neck, anterior chest wall
- Risk factors
  - Young age, active lifestyle, male gender, not cervical/first ribs
- Management
  - Diagnosis
    - Physical exam
      - Upper extremity swelling, cyanosis
      - Rule-out upper extremity phlegmasia
    - Duplex ultrasound
    - CT/MR venogram
    - Conventional venogram

        - May require positional imaging
  - Treatment
    - Initial management
      - Anticoagulation
    - Surgical options
      - Catheter-directed TPA
        - ✓ Indicated for acute thrombosis
    - Thoracic outlet decompression
        - ✓ First rib resection, anterior scalenectomy
        - ✓ Possible vein reconstruction with patch angioplasty
        - ✓ Timing after TPA is controversial (immediate vs 6 weeks out)

Arterial Thoracic Outlet Syndrome (ATOS)

- Etiology
  - Subclavian artery compression due to congenital or acquired bony abnormalities
    - Congenital deformities include prominent C7 TP (most common), cervical rib (2nd most common)
    - Acquired deformities include prior clavicle or first rib fracture
  - Stenosis and post-stenotic aneurysmal degeneration can cause thromboembolization
  - Intimal damage can be source of local arterial occlusion
  - 1% of TOS
- Presentation
  - Asymptomatic
  - Symptomatic with symptoms of limb ischemia (>50%)
    - Acute limb ischemia due to thromboembolism

        - Intermittent claudication due to positional arterial stenosis
    - Unilateral Raynaud syndrome
- Classification (Scher)
    - Stage 0: asymptomatic compression
    - Stage 1: post-stenotic dilatation
    - Stage 2: subclavian mural thrombus with intimal damage
    - Stage 3: distal embolization
- Risk factors
    - Cervical rib or abnormal first rib, prior clavicle fractures
- Management
    - Diagnosis
        - Physical exam
            - Elevated arm stress test (EAST): open and close hands in “surrender” position for three minutes
            - Blood pressure differential between arms
        - Duplex ultrasound
        - Chest X-ray
            - Cervical rib or abnormal first rib
        - CT angiogram
    - Treatment
        - Initial management
            - Anticoagulation
        - Surgical options
            - Catheter-directed thrombolysis
                - ✓ Indicated for acute thrombosis
            - Open embolectomy
                - ✓ Indicated for acute embolism

- Thoracic outlet decompression
  - ✓ First rib resection, anterior scalenectomy
  - ✓ Subclavian artery resection with interposition graft
- Indications for surgery
  - ✓ Scher stage 2/3

Pectoralis Minor Syndrome

- Etiology
  - o Brachial plexus compression within subcoracoid space
- Presentation
  - o Similar to neurogenic TOS symptoms
- Anatomy
  - o Pectoralis minor connects coracoid process to ribs 3-5
  - o Brachial plexus crosses underneath pectoralis minor at insertion into coracoid process
- Management
  - o Diagnosis
    - ▪ Physical exam (gold standard)
      - – Subcoracoid space tenderness, exacerbation of symptoms with palpation
      - – Relief of symptoms with pectoralis major contraction (distinguish from general muscle tenderness)
  - o Treatment
    - ▪ Surgical options
      - – Pectoralis minor tenotomy

Aberrant Right Subclavian Artery (Arteria Lusoria)

- Etiology
  - Right subclavian artery originates distal to left subclavian origin
    - Crosses midline between esophagus and spine
    - Associated anomalies include common carotid trunk, nonrecurrent laryngeal nerve, right-sided thoracic duct
  - Kommerell diverticulum: large posteromedial diverticulum at origin of artery
    - 0.5% prevalence
- Presentation
  - Asymptomatic
  - Symptomatic
    - Dysphagia lusoria (esophageal compression)
    - Acute limb ischemia (thromboembolism)
    - Respiratory distress in kids (tracheal compression)
    - Ortner syndrome: hoarseness (recurrent laryngeal nerve compression)
- Management
  - Diagnosis
    - CT/MR angiogram
  - Treatment
    - Surgical options
      - Right carotid-subclavian bypass with proximal subclavian ligation
      - Descending thoracic aortic replacement under DHCA
    - Indications for surgery
      - Symptoms, aneurysmal dilation >5.0 cm, Kommerell diverticulum >2.0 cm

Subclavian Artery Aneurysm

- Etiology
  - Subclavian artery diameter >150% normal
  - Multiple etiologies
    - Proximal subclavian aneurysms most commonly due to atherosclerosis
    - Distal subclavian aneurysms most commonly due to TOS
    - Other causes include trauma, connective tissue disorders, FMD, dissection
- Presentation
  - Asymptomatic (most common)
  - Symptomatic
    - Acute limb ischemia (thromboembolism)
    - Neck and upper extremity pain (mass effect)
    - Hemothorax (rupture, extremely rare)
- Anatomy
  - First segment is medial to anterior scalene
    - Internal mammary artery, vertebral artery, thyrocervical trunk
  - Second segment is deep to anterior scalene
    - Superior intercostal artery, deep cervical artery
  - Third segment is lateral to anterior scalene
    - Dorsal scapular artery
    - Becomes axillary artery at lateral border of 1st rib
- Risk factors
  - Male gender
- Management
  - Diagnosis
    - Duplex ultrasound
    - CT angiogram (gold standard)

    - Conventional angiogram
  - Treatment
    - Surgical options
      - Aneurysm resection with interposition graft
      - Covered stent placement
        - ✓ Risk of stent fracture due to clavicle
        - ✓ Long-term results unknown
    - Indications for surgery
      - Diameter ≥ 200%, symptoms

AXILLARY ARTERY ANEURYSM

- Etiology
  - Axillary artery diameter >150% normal
  - Multiple etiologies
    - Trauma is most common cause, classically due to chronic use of crutches
    - Other causes include connective tissue disorders, FMD, dissection
- Presentation
  - Asymptomatic
  - Acute limb ischemia (thromboembolism)
- Anatomy
  - First segment is medial to pectoralis minor
  - Second segment is posterior to pectoralis minor
  - Third segment is lateral to pectoralis minor
    - Becomes brachial artery at inferior border of teres major
- Risk factors
  - Male gender, athletic, use of crutches
- Management
  - Diagnosis

        - Duplex ultrasound
        - CT angiogram (gold standard)
        - Conventional angiogram
    - Treatment
        - Surgical options
            - Aneurysmorrhaphy
                - ✓ Preferred over aneurysm resection due to adjacent nerves
            - Aneurysm resection with interposition graft
            - Covered stent placement
                - ✓ Long-term results unknown
        - Indications for surgery
            - Diameter ≥ 200%, symptoms

Hypothenar Hammer Syndrome (HHS)

- Etiology
    - Aneurysmal degeneration of ulnar artery due to repetitive hypothenar trauma (hamate bone)
    - Can result in thrombosis, occlusion, or distal embolization
- Presentation
    - Asymptomatic
    - Symptomatic with digital pain and cold intolerance, digital ischemia, Raynaud phenomenon
        - Majority of patients have dominant hand symptoms
        - Primarily affects 3rd-5th fingers, thumb is always spared
- Risk factors
    - Male gender (90%), occupational exposure
- Management
    - Diagnosis

        - Physical exam
            - Allen test (positive if occluded)
            - Hypothenar callus
        - Duplex ultrasound
        - Conventional angiogram (gold standard)
            - Aneurysm, occlusion, or "corkscrew" ulnar artery
    - Treatment
        - Surgical options
            - Catheter-directed TPA
                - ✓ Ideal for occlusions with significant ischemic symptoms
            - Aneurysmectomy with interposition vein graft.

Chapter 3

Aortoiliac Review

Overview

- Descending Thoracic Aortic Aneurysm (DTAA)
- Thoraco-abdominal Aortic Aneurysm (TAAA)
- Abdominal Aortic Aneurysm (AAA)
- Ruptured Abdominal Aortic Aneurysm
- Inflammatory Abdominal Aortic Aneurysm
- Infected (Mycotic) Abdominal Aortic Aneurysm
- Isolated Common Iliac Artery Aneurysm (CIAA)
- Arteriomegaly/Aneurysmosis
- Aortocaval Fistula
- Aortoenteric Fistula (AEF)
- Aortic Dissection
- Aortic Intramural Hematoma (IMH)
- Penetrating Aortic Ulcer (PAU)
- Aortoiliac Occlusive Disease (AIOD)
- Acute Aortic Occlusion
- Erectile Dysfunction (ED)
- Pediatric Abdominal Aortic Aneurysm

- Abdominal Aortic Coarctation
- Endovascular Leak (Endoleak)
- Aortic Endograft Migration
- Ischemic Colitis (Post-evar)
- Aortic Graft Infection
- Pelvic Ischemia (Post-evar)
- Spinal Cord Ischemia
- Abdominal Compartment Syndrome (ACS)
- Chyle Leak

DESCENDING THORACIC AORTIC ANEURYSM (DTAA)

- Etiology
  - Aortic diameter >3 cm or >150% above normal
  - Involves aorta from left subclavian artery to diaphragm
- Presentation
  - Asymptomatic
  - Symptomatic with mass effect (esophagus, trachea, vertebral body, recurrent laryngeal nerve), back pain, or rupture
- Risk factors
  - Atherosclerosis (hypertension, hyperlipidemia, smoking, male gender)
  - Chronic type B dissections, previous aortic surgery, syphilis, trauma, connective tissue disorders (Marfan syndrome, Ehlers-Danlos syndrome, Loeys-Dietz syndrome)
- Management
  - Diagnosis
    - CT angiogram
    - Echocardiogram

- Treatment
  - Surgical options
    - Open aneurysm repair
      - ✓ Requires PFTs for single lung ventilation
      - ✓ Ideal for connective tissue disorders
    - TEVAR
      - ✓ 2 cm proximal/distal landing zones
      - ✓ 10% oversizing based on diameter
      - ✓ L subclavian coverage requires revascularization
      - ✓ Higher risk of stroke and paraplegia without revascularization
  - Debranching procedure
    - Indicated based on proximal landing zone
    - If zone 2 (left subclavian) coverage →
      - ✓ Left carotid-subclavian bypass
      - ✓ Left subclavian ligation to prevent type II endoleak
      - ✓ Left carotid-subclavian transposition
    - If zone 1 (left common carotid) coverage →
      - ✓ Carotid-carotid-subclavian bypass
      - ✓ Left subclavian ligation to prevent type II endoleak
      - ✓ Right carotid-left subclavian bypass with left carotid implantation
    - If zone 0 (innominate) coverage →
      - ✓ Aorto-innominate bypass with left carotid transposition and left carotid-subclavian bypass
    - Spinal cord protection
      - ✓ CSF drainage (<10 mmHg), hypothermia, neural monitoring, pressors (MAP >85 mmHg)
    - Indications for surgery

- ✓ Symptomatic aneurysms, size >5.5 cm, growth >1 cm/yr
- ✓ Lower threshold for connective tissue disorders (no size consensus)

Thoracoabdominal Aortic Aneurysm (TAAA)

- Etiology
  - Aortic diameter >3 cm or >150% above normal
  - Involves aorta from left subclavian artery to aortic bifurcation
- Presentation
  - Asymptomatic
  - Symptomatic with mass effect (esophagus, trachea, vertebral body, recurrent laryngeal nerve), back pain, or rupture
- Classification (Crawford)
  - Extent I: L subclavian to above renal arteries
  - Extent II: L subclavian to below renal arteries
  - Extent III: T6 to below renal arteries
  - Extent IV: T12 to below renal arteries
  - Extent V: T6 to above renal arteries
- Risk factors
  - Atherosclerosis (hypertension, hyperlipidemia, smoking, diabetes, male gender), syphilis, trauma
  - Connective tissue disorders (Marfan syndrome, Ehlers-Danlos syndrome, Loeys-Dietz syndrome)
    - 20% are associated with genetic syndrome
- Management
  - Diagnosis
    - CT angiogram

        - Echocardiogram
    - Treatment
        - Surgical options
            - Open aneurysm repair
                - ✓ Requires PFTs for single lung ventilation
                - ✓ Ideal for connective tissue disorders
            - FEVAR
            - Spinal cord protection
        - Indications for surgery
            - Symptomatic aneurysms, size >5.5 cm, growth >1 cm/yr
            - Lower threshold for connective tissue disorders (no size consensus)

ABDOMINAL AORTIC ANEURYSM (AAA)

- Etiology
    - Aortic diameter >3 cm or >150% normal
    - Complex process involving multiple factors
        - Elastin fragmentation within aortic wall
        - Chronic transmural inflammation
        - Dysregulated matrix metalloproteinases (MMP-9)
        - Smooth muscle cell ischemia due to lack of vasa vasorum
- Presentation
    - Asymptomatic found on screening ultrasound or other imaging
    - Asymptomatic pulsatile abdominal mass
    - Symptomatic with thrombosis, compression of adjacent organs, aortic dissection, rupture, embolization of mural debris

- Classification (anatomic)
    - Infrarenal: aneurysm doesn't involve renal arteries (97%)
    - Pararenal: aneurysm involves renal arteries (3%)
        - Juxtarenal: aneurysm neck <1 cm from renal arteries
        - Suprarenal: aneurysm above renal arteries but no visceral involvement
- Risk factors
    - Atherosclerosis (hypertension, hyperlipidemia, smoking, male gender), first-degree relatives (20% risk), ciprofloxacin
    - Connective tissue disorders (Marfan syndrome, Ehlers-Danlos syndrome, Loeys-Dietz syndrome)
    - Diabetes is paradoxically protective of AAA prevalence, growth, and rupture rate
- Management
    - Diagnosis
        - Abdominal ultrasound
            - Measure outer wall to outer wall
        - CT/MR angiogram
            - Evaluate for renal anomalies
                - ✓ Horseshoe kidney
                - ✓ Crossed renal ectopia
            - Evaluate for LRV anomalies
                - ✓ Retroaortic LRV (2%)
                - ✓ Circumaortic LRV or venous collar (8.7%)
            - Evaluate for IVC anomalies
                - ✓ Left-sided or transposed IVC (<1%)
                - ✓ Duplicate IVC (<3%)
    - Treatment
        - Medical management
            - Aspirin, smoking cessation, exercise, healthy diet

    - Treat hypertension (<140/90), diabetes (A1c <7%), hyperlipidemia (LDL <100 or <70 for diabetics)
  - Surgical options
    - Open aneurysm repair
    - EVAR
      - ✓ Lower 30-day mortality vs open repair but long-term survival is equivalent
      - ✓ Higher cost, need for long-term monitoring, higher rates of delayed interventions
      - ✓ Requires favorable anatomy (neck >15 mm, diameter <30 mm, angulation <60°, CFA >8 mm)
    - FEVAR
      - ✓ Ideal for pararenal or suprarenal aneurysms
  - Indications for surgery
    - Symptomatic aneurysms, size >5.5 cm (men) or >5.0 cm (women), growth >1 cm/yr, saccular aneurysms
- Screening
  - Abdominal ultrasound
    - Indicated for smoking men and women >65 years
  - If 3.0-3.9 cm → repeat 3 years
  - If 4.0-4.9 cm → repeat 1 year
  - If 5.0-5.4 cm → repeat 6 months

RUPTURED ABDOMINAL AORTIC ANEURYSM (RAAA)

- Etiology
  - Weakening of aneurysmal aorta results in tear in aortic wall
- Presentation

- Triad of hypotension, “tearing” abdominal/back pain, pulsatile abdominal mass
- >90% mortality rate

- Risk factors
  - Risk of rupture primarily related to aortic diameter
    - 5-6 cm has 10% annual risk of rupture
    - 6-7 cm has 15-20% annual risk of rupture
    - >7 cm has 30% annual risk of rupture
  - Other risks of rupture include saccular aneurysms, female gender, smoking/COPD, hypertension, ciprofloxacin
  - Diabetes is paradoxically protective of AAA prevalence, growth, and rupture rate
- Management
  - Diagnosis
    - CT angiogram (if stable)
    - No imaging necessary (if unstable)
  - Treatment
    - Initial management
      - Large bore IV access, blood transfusion, permissive hypotension
    - Surgical options
      - Open aneurysm repair
      - EVAR
        - ✓ Lower 30-day mortality vs open repair for rAAA

Inflammatory Abdominal Aortic Aneurysm

- Etiology
  - 5-10% of all AAAs are inflammatory type
  - Poorly understood process with multiple theories

        - Severe variant of AAA
        - Generalized autoimmune process with retroperitoneal fibrosis
        - *IgG4*-related autoimmune process
- Presentation
    - Back/flank pain, systemic symptoms (fever, weight loss, malaise), ureteral obstruction
        - 80-90% are symptomatic on presentation
    - Lower risk of rupture compared to non-inflammatory variant
- Risk factors
    - Similar risk factors as AAA but with several differences
    - Younger age (5-10 years), smokers, male gender
- Management
    - Diagnosis
        - Physical exam
            - Tender, pulsatile abdominal mass
        - CT/MR angiogram
            - Anterolateral wall thickening with sparing of posterior wall
            - Periaortic fibrosis involving duodenum, IVC, left renal vein, ureters
    - Treatment
        - Surgical options
            - Open aneurysm repair
                - ✓ Consider ureteral stenting prior to open repair
                - ✓ No randomized trial comparing outcomes between two procedures
            - EVAR
        - Indications for surgery
            - All inflammatory aneurysms

Infected (Mycotic) Abdominal Aortic Aneurysm

- Etiology
  - Multiple etiologies with similar endpoint
    - Hematogenous spread to normal or atherosclerotic aorta causes aneurysmal degeneration
    - Hematogenous spread to aortic aneurysm
    - Contiguous spread of adjacent site of infection
  - Bacterial growth within aortic wall causes destruction, dilatation, and eventual rupture
  - Organisms include *Staphylococcus* (most common), *Salmonella*, GNR, fungi
- Presentation
  - Abdominal/back pain, fever, leukocytosis, pulsatile abdominal mass
  - 50-85% rate of rupture
- Risk factors
  - Diabetes, catheter-based procedures, IV drug use, immunosuppression
- Management
  - Diagnosis
    - Physical exam
    - Tender, pulsatile abdominal mass
    - CT/MR angiogram
      - Periaortic inflammation (edema, fluid/gas), atypical location, saccular or multilobular shape
  - Treatment
    - Initial management
      - Blood cultures
      - IV antibiotics
    - Surgical options
      - Open repair

- Excise aneurysm, debride tissue, send for culture
- Aortic reconstruction (multiple options)
  - ✓ Axillo-bifemoral bypass
  - ✓ *In situ* reconstruction
  - ✓ Autogenous femoral vein graft
  - ✓ Cryopreserved homograft
  - ✓ Rifampin-soaked Dacron graft
- EVAR
  - ✓ Useful as bridge to definitive repair
  - ✓ Disadvantage is inability to debride infected tissue

▪ Indications for surgery
  - All mycotic aneurysms

ISOLATED COMMON ILIAC ARTERY ANEURYSM (CIAA)

- Etiology
  - Common iliac artery diameter >1.5 cm or >150% normal
  - Most common etiology is atherosclerotic degeneration
- Presentation
  - Asymptomatic (incidental finding)
  - Symptomatic with rupture or mass effect (groin/flank discomfort, ureteral obstruction, painful defecation, nerve compression)
- Classification (Sandhu)
  - Type A: CIAA with proximal neck and distal neck (≥1.5 cm)
  - Type B: CIAA with proximal neck, extends to bifurcation
  - Type C: CIAA with proximal neck, extends past bifurcation
  - Type D: isolated IIAA

- Type E: CIAA without proximal neck, bilateral CIAA, or CIAA with AAA
- Risk factors
  - Risk of rupture primarily related to CIAA diameter
    - <3 cm expands at 1 mm/year
    - >3 cm expands at 2.6 mm/year
- Management
  - Diagnosis
    - CT/MR angiogram
    - Conventional angiogram
  - Treatment
    - Surgical options
      - Open aneurysm repair
        - ✓ Consider ureteral stenting (13% injury rate)
      - Iliac covered stenting
        - ✓ 15 mm proximal/distal landing zones
        - ✓ May need IIA embolization to prevent endoleak
      - Iliac branch device insertion
    - Indications for surgery
      - Symptomatic aneurysms, size >3.5 cm (standalone) or >3.0 cm (if undergoing AAA repair)

ARTERIOMEGALY/ANEURYSMOSIS

- Etiology
  - Arteriomegaly: diffuse ectasia involving multiple arterial segments
  - Aneurysmosis: arteriomegaly complicated by aneurysmal degeneration
    - True cause of arteriomegaly and aneurysmosis is unknown

- Presentation
  - Asymptomatic
  - Symptomatic with thromboembolic complications (e.g., popliteal thrombosis)
- Classification (Hollier)
  - Type I: aortoiliac aneurysms
  - Type II: femoropopliteal aneurysms
  - Type III: both types I and II
    - >80% have type III aneurysmosis
- Management
  - Diagnosis
    - CT/MR angiogram
    - Conventional angiogram
  - Treatment
    - Open repair
      - Aneurysm resection with interposition graft
      - Staged repair for multiple aneurysms

AORTOCAVAL FISTULA

- Etiology
  - AAA fistulizes into adherent IVC
  - Combination of mechanical erosion and inflammation
  - Extremely rare (<1% incidence)
- Presentation
  - Abdominal bruits, pulsatile abdominal mass, abdominal/back pain, bilateral lower extremity edema
  - Severe tachycardia and heart failure due to increased preload
  - Lower extremity ischemia in severe cases of steal syndrome
- Risk factors

    - Large AAAs (average diameter 11 cm)
- Management
    - Diagnosis
        - CT/MR angiogram
    - Treatment
        - Surgical options
            - Open aneurysm repair
                - ✓ Sponge sticks can help with proximal/distal IVC control
                - ✓ Avoid IVC dissection due to friability
                - ✓ Fistula defect oversewn from within aneurysm sac
            - EVAR
                - ✓ Preferred over open repair due to blood loss
                - ✓ Risk of persistent type II endoleak, massive IVC thrombosis

Aortoenteric Fistula (AEF)

- Etiology
    - Primary AEF: AAA fistulizes into adherent GI tract through combination of mechanical erosion and inflammation
    - Secondary AEF: aortic graft fistulizes into adherent GI tract
        - 80% duodenum, 20% esophagus
- Presentation
    - Presents with hemorrhage, infection, or both
        - Small herald bleed (hematemesis) followed by massive GI bleed
        - Abdominal/back pain, fever, leukocytosis
- Management
    - Diagnosis

    - EGD
        - Mucosal erosion with adherent clot
        - Rule-out other causes of GI bleed
    - CT/MR angiogram
    - Tagged WBC scan
- Treatment
    - Initial management
        - NPO/NGT, IV antibiotics
    - Surgical options
        - Open aneurysm repair
            - ✓ Open aneurysm repair in standard fashion, debride tissue, send for culture
        - Duodenal repair
            - ✓ Primary repair vs resection/anastomosis
        - Aortic reconstruction (multiple options)
            - ✓ Axillo-bifemoral bypass
            - ✓ Autogenous femoral vein graft
            - ✓ Cryopreserved homograft
            - ✓ Rifampin-soaked Dacron graft
        - Covered stent insertion
            - ✓ Palliative option to temporize hemorrhage
- Prevention
    - Cover graft with aneurysm sac and omentum during open AAA repair

AORTIC DISSECTION

- Etiology
    - Intimal tear results in dissection of medial layers of aorta
    - False lumen can propagate, thrombose, or compromise branch perfusion

        - Static obstruction occurs when flap enters origin of branch artery
        - Dynamic obstruction occurs when flap covers origin of branch artery
- Presentation
    - Acute onset severe chest/back pain, unequal pulses, malperfusion
    - Uncomplicated dissection: no rupture, no malperfusion, no high-risk features
    - High-risk dissection: refractory pain, refractory hypertension, aortic diameter >40 mm
    - Complicated dissection: rupture and/or malperfusion
- Classification
    - Stanford classification
        - Type A: involves ascending aorta ± descending aorta
        - Type B: involves descending aorta only
    - DeBakey classification
        - Type I: involves both ascending and descending aorta
        - Type II: involves ascending aorta only
        - Type III: involves descending aorta only
    - SVS/STS classification
        - Anatomic location based on zones
    - Chronicity
        - Hyperacute <24 hrs
        - Acute 1-14 days
        - Subacute 15-90 days
        - Chronic >90 days
- Risk factors
    - Severe hypertension, trauma, syphilis, cocaine, male gender
    - Connective tissue disorders (Marfan syndrome, Ehlers-Danlos syndrome, Loeys-Dietz syndrome)
- Management

- Diagnosis
  - Chest X-ray
    - Abnormal aortic contour, wide mediastinum, pleural effusion, displaced intimal calcification, hemothorax
  - CT angiogram
  - Transesophageal echocardiogram
- Treatment
  - Initial management
    - Admit to ICU
    - Impulse control (HR 60-80, SBP 100-110), pain control
      - ✓ Esmolol gtt, nitroprusside gtt
  - If type A →
    - Emergent open repair
  - If type B →
    - Surgical options
      - ✓ TEVAR (first line)
        - ❖ 1.6% incidence of retrograde type A dissection
        - ❖ Risk factors include landing zone diameter >40 mm and oversizing graft >10%
    - Open aortic repair
    - Open aortic fenestration
    - Branch artery stenting
    - Branch artery bypass
      - ✓ Indicated for visceral malperfusion
    - Femoro-femoral bypass
      - ✓ Indicated for persistent lower extremity ischemia
    - Indications for surgery

  - ✓ Urgent indications: acute complicated dissection, high-risk features, connective tissue disorder
  - ✓ Elective indications: chronic dissection with aortic diameter >5.5 cm, growth >1 cm/year

AORTIC INTRAMURAL HEMATOMA (IMH)

- Etiology
  - Spontaneous rupture of vasa vasorum causes hemorrhage within aortic wall without intimal tear
  - Lacks direct communication between false and true lumen (compared to dissection)
- Presentation
  - Symptoms similar to aortic dissection
- Classification
  - Stanford classification
    - Type A IMH: involves ascending aorta ± descending aorta
    - Type B IMH: involves descending aorta only
  - SVS/STS classification
    - Anatomic location based on zones
- Management
  - Similar to aortic dissection

PENETRATING ATHEROSCLEROTIC ULCER (PAU)

- Etiology
  - Atherosclerotic ulcer that penetrates elastic lamina
  - Can progress to IMH, aortic dissection, and rupture

- Presentation
  - Symptoms similar to aortic dissection
- Classification
  - Stanford classification
    - Type A PAU: involves ascending aorta ± descending aorta
    - Type B PAU: involves descending aorta only
  - SVS/STS classification
    - Anatomic location based on zones
- Management
  - Similar to aortic dissection

AORTOILIAC OCCLUSIVE DISEASE (AIOD)

- Etiology
  - Atherosclerotic plaques form in aorta and iliac arteries
  - Plaques become clinically significant due to stenosis, occlusion, or embolization
- Presentation
  - Asymptomatic (50%)
  - Atypical leg pain (30%)
  - Intermittent claudication (15%)
  - Chronic limb-threatening ischemia (<5%)
    - Rest pain or tissue loss
    - Symptom duration >2 weeks
- Classification (Rutherford)
  - Category 0: asymptomatic
  - Category 1: mild claudication
  - Category 2: moderate claudication
  - Category 3: severe claudication
  - Category 4: ischemic rest pain

    - Category 5: minor tissue loss
    - Category 6: major tissue loss
- Risk factors
    - Atherosclerosis (hypertension, hyperlipidemia, smoking, diabetes, male gender)
- Management
    - Diagnosis
        - Physical exam
        - Arterial LENIs
            - ABI/PVRs
                - ✓ >1.3 indicates calcified vessels
                - ✓ 0.9-1.3 is normal
                - ✓ 0.4-0.9 indicates claudication
                - ✓ <0.4 indicates rest pain
            - Exercise treadmill testing
                - ✓ Indicated for claudicants with normal ABIs
                - ✓ Drop of 25 mmHg that persists >2 minutes is abnormal
            - Toe pressures
                - ✓ >40 mmHg indicates good healing potential (>60 mmHg in diabetics)
        - CT/MR angiogram
        - Conventional angiogram (gold standard)
    - Treatment
        - Medical management
            - Aspirin, smoking cessation, exercise, healthy diet
            - Treat hypertension (<140/90), diabetes (A1c <7%), hyperlipidemia (LDL <100 or <70 for diabetics)
            - First-line therapy for intermittent claudication and asymptomatic disease
                - ✓ Only 5% of claudicants progress to limb loss in 5 years

- Surgical options
  - Aorto-bifemoral bypass (gold standard)
    - ✓ End-to-end proximal anastomosis advantageous with less competitive flow, better hemodynamic configuration, less likely to develop distal atheroembolization, easier to cover with retroperitoneal tissue
    - ✓ End-to-side proximal anastomosis preferred for patent IMA, infrarenal accessory renal artery, bilateral EIA occlusive disease with poor retrograde flow to IIA
  - Aortic endarterectomy
    - ✓ Ideal for focal aortic lesions
  - Ilio-femoral bypass
    - ✓ Ideal for focal EIA lesions
  - Axillo-bifemoral bypass
    - ✓ Ideal for poor surgical candidates
  - Angioplasty/stenting
- Indications for surgery
  - Critical limb ischemia, lifestyle-limiting claudication

ACUTE AORTIC OCCLUSION

- Etiology
  - Acute occlusion of the infrarenal aorta
  - Most common causes are cardiogenic emboli or *in situ* thrombosis
    - Cardiogenic emboli lodge at aortic bifurcation with retrograde propagation

        - *In situ* thrombosis of severe AIOD often precipitated by dehydration or MI
        - Rare causes include dissection, hypercoagulable state, HITT, trauma, graft thrombosis
- Presentation
    - Severe pain (primary symptom), pulselessness, lower extremity neurologic deficits
    - Skin pallor, mottling, cyanosis extending to level of umbilicus
    - Revascularization can cause significant reperfusion injury and multisystem organ failure
- Management
    - Diagnosis
        - CT angiogram
    - Treatment
        - Initial management
            - Anticoagulation, fluid resuscitation
            - Invasive hemodynamic monitoring
        - Surgical options
            - Bilateral transfemoral thromboembolectomy
                - ✓ Ideal for embolic disease
            - Aorto-bifemoral bypass
            - Axillo-bifemoral bypass
            - Angioplasty/stenting
                - ✓ Ideal for *in situ* thrombosis
            - Bilateral fasciotomies
                - ✓ Indicated for prolonged ischemia time (>4-6 hrs)

ERECTILE DYSFUNCTION (ED)

- Etiology
  - Vasculogenic ED: atherosclerotic obstruction or endothelial dysfunction of penile arteries
  - Neurogenic ED: iatrogenic injury to pelvic nerves or diabetic dysautonomia
    - 90% of cases are organic due to underlying anatomic problems
  - Psychogenic ED: failure to achieve ED due to non-anatomic causes
    - 10% of cases are psychogenic and respond well to placebo therapy
- Presentation
  - Recurrent or persistent inability to attain/maintain erection
    - Must result in lack of satisfactory sexual activity for 3 months
  - ED is a marker of significantly increased risk of CV disease
    - Precedes onset of other CV events by 2-5 years
    - Often the first manifestation of generalized condition
- Anatomy
  - Arterial blood supply to penis
    - Internal iliac → internal pudendal → common penile artery
    - Common penile branches into dorsal penile and deep (central) penile arteries
      - Dorsal penile artery supplies skin and glans of penis
      - Deep penile artery supplies corpus cavernosum, responsible for erection
  - Innervation of penile function
    - Parasympathetic nerves control erection
    - Sympathetic nerves control ejaculation

- Risk factors
    - Atherosclerosis (hypertension, hyperlipidemia, smoking, diabetes)
- Management
    - Diagnosis
        - Clinical diagnosis
        - Full medical evaluation
            - All ED patients mandate full medical assessment including baseline activity (Princeton guidelines)
    - Treatment
        - Medical management
            - Aspirin, smoking cessation, exercise, healthy diet
        - If organic →
            - PDE5 inhibitors (sildenafil, vardenafil, tadalafil)
                - ✓ First-line treatment
                - ✓ Contraindicated with nitrites
            - Alprostadil (PGE1)
                - ✓ Intracavernosal injection
                - ✓ Urethral suppository
            - Testosterone therapy
                - ✓ For documented low levels only
            - Vacuum constriction devices
            - Penile implants
                - ✓ Last-line invasive option
        - If psychogenic →
            - Psychotherapy

PEDIATRIC ABDOMINAL AORTIC ANEURYSM

- Etiology
    - Abnormal dilation of aorta in pediatric patient

- Majority are saccular (compared to fusiform in adults)
- Multiple etiologies including infectious, genetic, idiopathic, or post-traumatic
  - Infection most commonly due to umbilical artery catheterization
  - Genetic causes include Marfan, Ehlers-Danlos vascular type, tuberculous sclerosis
  - Idiopathic AAA includes post-stenotic turbulent flow with aortic coarctation

- Presentation
  - Asymptomatic pulsatile abdominal mass
  - Symptomatic with thrombosis, compression of adjacent organs, aortic dissection, rupture, embolization of mural debris
- Management
  - Diagnosis
    - CT/MR angiogram
    - Conventional angiogram
  - Treatment
    - Surgical options
      - Aneurysmectomy with interposition graft
        - ✓ Use the largest diameter graft as safely possible
        - ✓ Options include aorto-aortic or aorto-iliac grafting
      - Endovascular repair suboptimal due to child outgrowing endograft

Abdominal Aortic Coarctation

- Etiology
  - Aortic diameter <50% normal secondary to hypoplasia

  - Likely due to defective "overfusion" of two primitive dorsal aortas
- Presentation
  - Asymptomatic
  - Symptoms vary with level of coarctation
    - Suprarenal lesions present with triad of severe hypertension, absent femoral pulses, abdominal bruits
      - Average age of symptom onset is 10-20 yo
    - Infrarenal lesions present with lower extremity fatigue and intermittent claudication
      - Average age of symptom onset is 40-50 yo
- Classification (anatomic)
  - Suprarenal coarctation: 70%, most superior narrowing cephalad to renal arteries
  - Pararenal coarctation: 20%, most superior narrowing at level of renal arteries
  - Infrarenal coarctation: 10%, most superior narrowing caudal to renal arteries
- Risk factors
  - Female gender, red hair
  - Genetic syndromes (Turner syndrome, Williams syndrome, neurofibromatosis type I)
- Management
  - Diagnosis
    - CT/MR angiogram
    - Conventional angiogram
  - Treatment
    - Surgical options
      - Patch aortoplasty (gold standard)
      - Thoraco-abdominal bypass
        - ✓ Indicated when coarcted aorta is too small to patch

- Aorto-bifemoral bypass
  - ✓ Indicated for symptomatic infrarenal coarctation complicated by atherosclerosis
- Endovascular repair not recommended due to high incidence of early restenosis

ENDOVASCULAR LEAK (ENDOLEAK)

- Etiology
  - Persistent bloodflow within aneurysm sac after endovascular repair
- Presentation
  - Asymptomatic sac expansion on surveillance imaging
  - Symptomatic with mass effect or rupture after EVAR
- Classification
  - Type I endoleak
    - Incomplete seal at proximal (Ia) or distal (Ib) graft
    - Early type I considered failure of procedure (typically for devices outside of IFU)
    - Delayed type I occur due to graft migration, aneurysmal degeneration of aortic neck or iliac arteries
  - Type II endoleak
    - Branch vessel fills sac in retrograde fashion
    - Caused by patent lumbar arteries, IMA, or internal iliacs
    - Majority (>2/3) resolve spontaneously by 6 months
  - Type III endoleak
    - Junctional defect between graft components (IIIa) or fabric holes (IIIb)
  - Type IV endoleak
    - Early graft porosity that typically resolves within 24 hours

        - May obscure type I or III endoleaks
    - Type V endoleak
        - "Endotension", continued sac expansion without leak on imaging
        - Possibly due to protein-rich exudate from original e-PTFE endografts
- Management
    - Diagnosis
        - CT/MR angiogram
        - Conventional angiogram
    - Treatment
        - If type I →
            - Graft explantation with open AAA repair
                - ✓ Best option for good surgical candidates
            - Proximal aortic cuff (need favorable aortic neck)
            - Aorto-uni-iliac grafting with femoral-femoral bypass
            - Endovascular screws (*Aptus EndoAnchor*®)
        - If type II →
            - Observation (6 months)
            - Transarterial embolization
            - Translumbar embolization
            - Open ligation
        - If type III →
            - Stent grafting (seals fabric defect or disjoined modular components)
        - If type IV →
            - Observation
        - Indications for surgery
            - All type I and III, persistent type II (>6 months)

AORTIC ENDOGRAFT MIGRATION

- Etiology
  - Two definitions
    - Caudal movement >10 mm
    - Caudal movement with symptoms
  - Can occur anytime but average interval is 3-4 years
- Presentation
  - Asymptomatic finding during surveillance imaging
  - Symptomatic with type Ia endoleak
- Risk factors
  - Aortic neck anatomy (length <15 mm, angulation >60°, conical morphology)
  - Endograft oversizing >30%, delayed aortic neck degeneration, non-fixed endografts (*AneuRx*®)
- Management
  - Diagnosis
    - CT/MR angiogram
    - Conventional angiogram
  - Treatment
    - Surgical options
      - Graft explantation with open AAA repair
        - ✓ Best option for good surgical candidates
      - Proximal aortic cuff (need favorable aortic neck)
      - Aorto-uni-iliac grafting with femoral-femoral bypass
      - Endovascular screws (*Aptus EndoAnchor*®)

Ischemic Colitis (Post-EVAR)

- Etiology
    - Colonic ischemia due to exclusion or ligation of IMA
- Presentation
    - LLQ abdominal pain, bloody diarrhea, fever, leukocytosis
- Risk factors
    - Previous colonic or retroperitoneal surgery (impacts left colon perfusion)
- Management
    - Diagnosis
        - Flexible sigmoidoscopy
    - Treatment
        - Medical management
            - NPO/NGT, fluid resuscitation
            - IV antibiotics
        - Surgical options
            - Sigmoid colectomy
        - Indications for surgery
            - Peritonitis, transmural ischemia on endoscopy
    - Prevention
        - Open AAA repair with IMA reimplantation (avoid EVAR)
        - Indicated for isolated left colon perfusion from patent IMA

Aortic Graft Infection

- Etiology
    - Bacterial infection of aortic graft after AIOD or AAA repair

  - Organisms include *S. aureus* (most common), *S. epidermidis, Pseudomonas*, GNR
- Presentation
  - Early graft infections more likely to have systemic symptoms
    - Abdominal/back pain, fever, leukocytosis, sepsis
  - Late graft infections more likely to have a more indolent presentation
    - Groin wound infection, abscess, draining sinus tract
  - Can also be a manifestation of secondary aortoenteric fistula or erosion
- Risk factors
  - Emergent procedures, femoral anastomosis
- Management
  - Diagnosis
    - CT angiogram
    - Sinography
      - Inject sinus tract with contrast to determine extent of graft involvement
      - Hypothetical risk of spreading infection to uninvolved graft
    - Tagged WBC scan
    - FDG-PET scan
  - Treatment
    - Medical management
      - IV antibiotics
    - Surgical options
      - Graft explantation, debride tissue, send for culture
      - Revascularization (multiple options)
        - ✓ Axillo-bifemoral bypass (traditional)
        - ✓ Autogenous femoral vein graft (preferred)

- ✓ Need 5 mm femoral veins without thrombus or sclerosis
- ✓ Venous morbidity is uncommon after vein harvest (15%)
- – Cryopreserved allograft
  - ✓ High cost and limited availability
- – Rifampin-soaked Dacron graft
  - ✓ Rifampin has broad-spectrum activity, low resistance profile, sticks to graft due to hydrophobic nature
  - ✓ Consider for low-grade biofilm (*S. epidermidis*)

Pelvic Ischemia (Post-EVAR)

- Etiology
  - o 10-40% risk of pelvic ischemia with embolization/ligation of IIA
  - o Embolization may be needed to prevent type II endoleak with CIA aneurysms
  - o Increased risk with simultaneous bilateral IIA occlusion
- Presentation
  - o Buttock claudication (most common)
  - o Other symptoms include colonic ischemia, spinal cord ischemia, pelvic necrosis, erectile dysfunction
  - o Severe pelvic ischemia can lead to gluteal necrosis, perineal necrosis, bladder/rectal dysfunction
- Risk factors
  - o Pelvic radiation, heart failure (low flow), diffuse atherosclerotic disease

- Angiographic predictors include >70% stenosis of contralateral IIA, non-opacification of 3+ IIA branches, diseased/absent ipsilateral PFA

- Management
  - Diagnosis
    - Clinical diagnosis
    - CT/MR angiogram
    - Conventional angiogram
  - Treatment
    - Supportive care
  - Prevention
    - Selective proximal embolization
      - Occlude main trunk and leave anterior/posterior branches patent
      - Preserve collaterals from femoral and external iliac arteries
    - Staged bilateral embolization (if needed)
      - Allows development of collateral flow
    - Open IIA reimplantation
    - Endovascular iliac branch device (IBD)

Spinal Cord Ischemia

- Etiology
  - Interruption of intercostal/lumbar blood flow by aortic occlusion
  - Occurs with both open (more common) and endovascular repair
  - Highest risk with covering T8-L1 segments
- Presentation

  - Urinary/fecal incontinence, sensorimotor deficits, flaccid paralysis of bilateral lower extremities
  - Maximal risk at 48-72 hrs post-op
- Classification (Modified Tarlov scale)
  - Rank 0: no motor function
  - Rank 1: lift leg but not against gravity
  - Rank 2: lift leg against gravity
  - Rank 3: stand with assistance
  - Rank 4: walk with assistance
  - Rank 5: walk without assistance
- Risk factors
  - Length of aortic coverage
    - Extent I (15%), extent II (31%), extent III (7%), extent IV (4%)
    - Percentages from the "clamp and sew" era
  - Hypotension, anemia, CKD (low GFR)
  - Left subclavian coverage without revascularization
- Management
  - Diagnosis
    - Physical exam
    - MRI spine
    - Rule-out paraspinal hematoma
  - Treatment
    - Optimize spinal cord perfusion
      - MAP >90 mmHg
      - CSF pressure <10 mmHg
      - Hgb >10 g/dL
  - Prevention
    - Hypothermia (32-34°C)
    - Neural monitoring (somatosensory and motor-evoked potentials)

        - Intercostal reimplantation
        - Lumbar spinal drainage

ABDOMINAL COMPARTMENT SYNDROME (ACS)

- Etiology
    - Increased intraabdominal pressure (IAP) often seen in the setting of ruptured AAA and massive resuscitation
- Presentation
    - Increased peak pressures (diaphragm compression)
    - Decreased cardiac output (IVC compression reduces preload)
    - Acute kidney injury (renal vein compression)
    - Intestinal edema (mesenteric vein compression)
- Classification (WSACS)
    - Intra-abdominal hypertension (IAH)
        - IAH grade I: IAP 12-15 mmHg
        - IAH grade II: IAP 16-20 mmHg
        - IAH grade III: IAP 21-25 mmHg
        - IAH grade IV: IAP ≥26 mmHg
    - Abdominal compartment syndrome (ACS)
        - ACS: IAP ≥20 mmHg with end-organ dysfunction
        - Primary ACS: ACS related to abdominopelvic process
        - Secondary ACS: ACS not related to abdominopelvic process
        - Recurrent ACS: ACS redevelops after initial treatment
- Management
    - Diagnosis
        - Bladder pressure
            - Fill with 25 ml of sterile saline
            - Transduce through three-way Foley while paralyzed

        - All ruptured AAA require IAH surveillance
    - Intragastric pressure
        - Alternative when Foley is contraindicated
- Treatment
    - Medical management
        - NPO/NGT
        - Sedation/analgesia
        - Paralysis
    - Surgical options
        - Decompressive laparotomy
    - Indications for surgery
        - End-organ dysfunction, refractory intra-abdominal hypertension

Chyle Leak

- Etiology
    - Injury to lymphatic channels or thoracic duct during aortic repair
    - Results in development of chyloperitoneum (chylous ascites) or chylothorax
- Presentation
    - Chyloperitoneum: early satiety, abdominal distention, nausea/emesis
    - Chylothorax: shortness of breath, pleural effusion
- Anatomy
    - Cisterna chyli forms posterolateral to right of aorta
        - Ascends into pleural cavity at L1 level, becoming thoracic duct
    - Thoracic duct crosses from right to left retropleural space at T4/T5 level

        - Empties into left SC/IJ junction, 2-3 cm above left clavicle
    - Right lymphatic duct empties into right SC/IJ junction above right clavicle
    - Lots of anatomic variability (~50%)
- Management
    - Diagnosis
        - CT scan
            - Ascites or pleural effusion
        - Diagnostic paracentesis
        - Diagnostic thoracentesis
            - Triglyceride levels (>110 mg/dL), chylomicrons, lymphocytes, milky fluid
        - Lymphoscintigraphy
    - Treatment
        - Medical management
            - First-line therapy
            - High protein, low fat MCT diet
            - Bowel rest with TPN
            - Octreotide injections
        - Surgical options
            - Surgical thoracic duct ligation
                - ✓ Drinking high-fat cream before operation may help identify leak
            - Thoracic duct embolization
                - ✓ Reserved for high-risk patients
                - ✓ Not available at many institutions
            - Peritoneovenous shunt (Denver or LeVeen)

    - ✓ Legacy procedure due to high incidence of DIC and infection
- Indications for surgery
  - Persistent chyle leak refractory to conservative management

Chapter 4

LOWER EXTREMITY REVIEW

OVERVIEW

- Infrainguinal Occlusive Disease (IIOD)
- Bypass Graft Stenosis/Occlusion
- Acute Limb Ischemia (ALI)
- Persistent Sciatic Artery (PSA)
- Popliteal Artery Entrapment Syndrome (PAES)
- Adventitial Cystic Disease
- Diabetic Foot Ulcers (DFU)
- Femoral Artery Aneurysm (FAA)
- Infected Femoral Artery Pseudoaneurysm
- Popliteal Artery Aneurysm (PAA)
- Atheroembolism
- Extremity Compartment Syndrome

INFRAINGUINAL OCCLUSIVE DISEASE (IIOD)

- Etiology
  - Atherosclerotic plaques form in femoral, popliteal, and infrapopliteal arteries
  - Plaques become clinically significant due to stenosis, occlusion, or embolization
- Presentation
  - Asymptomatic (50%)
  - Atypical leg pain (30%)
  - Intermittent claudication (15%)
  - Critical limb ischemia (<5%)
    - Rest pain or tissue loss
    - Symptom duration >14 days
- Classification (Rutherford)
  - Category 0: asymptomatic
  - Category 1: mild claudication
  - Category 2: moderate claudication
  - Category 3: severe claudication
  - Category 4: ischemic rest pain
  - Category 5: minor tissue loss
  - Category 6: major tissue loss
- Risk factors
  - Atherosclerosis (hypertension, hyperlipidemia, smoking, diabetes, male gender)
- Management
  - Diagnosis
    - Physical exam
      - Rule-out neurogenic claudication
    - Arterial LENIs
      - ABI/PVRs
        - ✓ >1.3 indicates calcified vessels

- ✓ 0.9-1.3 is normal
- ✓ 0.4-0.9 indicates claudication
- ✓ <0.4 indicates rest pain

- – Exercise treadmill testing
  - ✓ Indicated for claudicants with normal ABIs
  - ✓ Drop of 25 mmHg that persists >2 minutes is abnormal
- – Toe pressures
  - ✓ >40 mmHg indicates good healing potential (>60 mmHg in diabetics)

- ▪ CT/MR angiogram
- ▪ Conventional angiogram (gold standard)
  - – Useful for bypass planning

- o Treatment
  - ▪ Medical management
    - – Aspirin, smoking cessation, exercise, healthy diet
    - – Treat hypertension (<140/90), diabetes (A1c <7%), hyperlipidemia (LDL <100 or <70 for diabetes)
    - – First-line therapy for intermittent claudication and asymptomatic disease
      - ✓ Only 5% of claudicants progress to limb loss in 5 years
  - ▪ Surgical options
    - – Bypass graft (gold standard)
      - ✓ Multiple conduit options
        - ❖ Ipsilateral GSV (reversed, non-reversed, in situ)
        - ❖ Contralateral GSV (reversed, non-reversed)
        - ❖ Short saphenous vein
        - ❖ Arm veins
        - ❖ Synthetic grafts (ePTFE, Dacron)
      - ✓ Patency rates vary with conduit and location

- ✓ Vein mapping
  - ❖ Need 3 mm vein without thrombotic or sclerotic segments
- – Femoral endarterectomy
  - ✓ Ideal for focal CFA lesions
  - ✓ Can be used in conjunction with endovascular procedures
- – Deep femoral angioplasty (profundaplasty)
  - ✓ Ideal for severe PFA stenosis with SFA occlusion
- – Angioplasty/stenting
  - ✓ Balloon angioplasty
  - ✓ Drug-coated balloon angioplasty
  - ✓ Bare-metal stents
  - ✓ Drug-eluting stents (paclitaxel, sirolimus)
    - ❖ Paclitaxel inhibits microtubules
  - ✓ Covered stents (Viabahn endograft)
    - ❖ Not recommended for popliteal or infrapopliteal lesions
  - ✓ Atherectomy
  - ✓ Cryoplasty
- – Amputation
  - ✓ Last resort option
  - ✓ Indicated for uncontrolled pain or uncontrolled infection

▪ Indications for surgery
- – Chronic limb-threatening ischemia, lifestyle-limiting claudication

- Studies
  - o BASIL trial: CLTI patients undergoing surgical bypass (vs angioplasty) have improved mortality and wound healing rates at 2-year follow-up

- COMPASS trial: PAD patients on ASA and Xarelto (2.5 mg BID) (vs ASA alone) have lower rates of stroke, amputation, and cardiovascular death

BYPASS GRAFT STENOSIS/OCCLUSION

- Etiology
  - Etiology depends on timing of stenosis or occlusion
    - <30 days indicates technical error
    - 30 days – 2 years due to neointimal hyperplasia
    - >2 years due to recurrent atherosclerosis
  - Location varies based on conduit type
    - GSV lesions – 70% within graft, 30% at proximal/distal anastomoses
    - PTFE lesions – 30% at proximal anastomosis, 60% distal anastomosis, <10% within graft
- Presentation
  - Asymptomatic (60%)
  - Intermittent claudication (30%)
  - Critical limb ischemia (10%)
- Risk factors
  - Patency depends conduit, location (above or below knee), indication (IC vs CLI)
  - Vein diameter <3 mm or non-single segment vein graft
  - Above knee
    - GSV primary patency rate 80% (1 yr) and 70% (5 yrs)
    - PTFE primary patency rate 80% (1 yr) and 70% (5 yrs)
  - Below knee
    - GSV primary patency rate 80% (1 yr) and 70% (5 yrs)
    - PTFE primary patency rate 60% (1 yr) and 20-40% (5 yrs)

- Management
  - Diagnosis
    - Duplex ultrasound
      - Impending graft failure: PSV <45 cm/sec
      - <50% stenosis: PSV <150 cm/sec, PSV ratio <2.0
      - 50-69% stenosis: PSV 150-300 cm/sec, PSV ratio 2.0-3.5
      - >70% stenosis: PSV >300 cm/sec, PSV ratio >3.5
    - CT/MR angiogram
    - Conventional angiogram
  - Treatment
    - Medical management
      - Aspirin, smoking cessation, exercise, healthy diet
      - Treat hypertension (<140/90), diabetes (A1c <7%), hyperlipidemia (LDL <100 or <70 for diabetics)
      - Anticoagulation
        - ✓ Indicated for low-flow grafts (PSV <45)
    - Surgical options
      - Open graft revision (gold standard)
        - ✓ Thrombectomy
        - ✓ Patch angioplasty
        - ✓ Graft excision with primary anastomosis
        - ✓ Graft excision with interposition graft
        - ✓ Distal jump grafting
      - Angioplasty
        - ✓ Indicated for focal stenosis (<2 cm) only
        - ✓ Not indicated for occlusions due to high early failure rates
      - Catheter-directed TPA
        - ✓ Indicated for acute graft thrombosis
    - Indications for surgery

    - >70% stenosis, early graft occlusions, symptomatic late graft occlusions
  - Screening
    - Graft duplex
      - ✓ 30 days, 6/12/18/24 mo, annual afterwards

ACUTE LIMB ISCHEMIA (ALI)

- Etiology
  - Sudden, critical reduction in extremity arterial blood flow
    - Irreversible damage occurs after 6 hrs
    - Revascularization results in reperfusion injury
  - Multiple etiologies – arterial embolism, acute on chronic thrombosis, traumatic occlusion, dissection, paradoxical embolism, popliteal artery aneurysm
    - Femoral bifurcation (50% of macroemboli)
    - Aortic bifurcation (35%)
    - Popliteal artery (<15%)
- Presentation
  - 6 Ps – pain, pallor, pulselessness, parasthesias, paralysis, poikilothermia
  - Symptom duration <14 days (as opposed to CLTI)
- Classification (Rutherford)
  - Category I: viable; no deficits
  - Category II: threatened; mild deficits
    - Category IIa: sensory deficits only
    - Category IIb: sensory and motor deficits
  - Category III: irreversible; complete sensory and motor loss
- Risk factors
  - Atrial fibrillation, recent myocardial infarction, prosthetic heart valves, endocarditis

- Management
  - Diagnosis
    - Duplex ultrasound
    - CT angiogram
    - Conventional angiogram
  - Treatment
    - Initial management
      - Anticoagulation
    - Surgical options
      - Open thromboembolectomy
        - ✓ Ideal for all embolic lesions, thrombotic lesions >14 days old
      - Catheter-directed TPA
        - ✓ Indicated for category I or IIa
        - ✓ Ideal for thrombotic lesions <14 days old with proper thrombus cannulation
        - ✓ Monitor fibrinogen levels (stop for <100 mg/dl)
        - ✓ Absolute contraindications include active bleeding, recurrent GI bleeding, recent intracranial or spinal operation, known intracranial pathologic lesion, uncontrolled severe hypertension
      - Percutaneous mechanical thrombectomy
      - Percutaneous suction thrombectomy
      - Lower extremity fasciotomy
        - ✓ Indicated for ischemic time >4-6 hrs
      - Amputation
        - ✓ Indicated for category III

Persistent Sciatic Artery (PSA)

- Etiology
  - Failure of regression of embryonal sciatic artery
    - Originates from IIA and continues as popliteal artery
    - Courses through greater sciatic foramen along adductor magnus
  - Rare (0.05% incidence) with 20% bilateral lesions
  - Prone to early atherosclerosis and aneurysmal degeneration due to repetitive hip extension/flexion
- Presentation
  - Asymptomatic (40%)
  - Symptomatic (60%)
    - Acute limb ischemia secondary to thromboembolism
    - Sciatic nerve compression with larger aneurysms
    - Severe gluteal pain and ecchymosis with aneurysm rupture
- Classification
  - Complete sciatic artery: 80%, PSA extends from IIA to popliteal artery, early SFA termination
  - Incomplete sciatic artery: 20%, PSA terminates early, SFA extends from EIA to popliteal artery
- Management
  - Diagnosis
    - Physical exam
      - Cowie sign: diminished femoral pulse with intact distal pulses
      - Pulsatile mass over buttock region
    - CT/MR angiogram
    - Conventional angiogram
  - Treatment
    - Surgical options

        - Open ligation (incomplete only)
        - Open ligation with femoro-popliteal bypass (complete)
        - Open aneurysmorrhaphy
        - Coil embolization (incomplete only)
        - Covered stent insertion
    - Indications for surgery
        - Symptomatic PSA, aneurysmal degeneration

Popliteal Artery Entrapment Syndrome (PAES)

- Etiology
    - Medial deviation of popliteal artery around medial head of gastrocnemius
- Presentation
    - Intermittent claudication in otherwise young, healthy patient
    - Loss of pulse with plantarflexion (compared to adventitial cystic disease)
- Classification
    - Type I: abnormal course of popliteal artery
    - Type II: abnormal position of nearby muscle
    - Type III: accessory slip of nearby muscle and fibrous bands of tissue
    - Type IV: popliteal artery passes underneath the popliteus muscle
    - Type V: compression of the popliteal artery/vein
    - Type VI: other variations
- Risk factors
    - Male gender, athletes
- Management
    - Diagnosis

        - Stress positional testing
            - ABI decrease by 30% with plantarflexion or dorsiflexion
            - MR angiogram (gold standard)
            - Evaluates muscles, tendons, vessels
    - Treatment
        - Surgical options
            - Resect medial head of gastrocnemius
        - Indications for surgery
            - Symptomatic PAES

Adventitial Cystic Disease

- Etiology
    - Single or multiloculated cysts located within adventitial layer
        - Most commonly found within popliteal artery
        - Also found rarely in EIA, CFA, radial, ulnar arteries
    - Mucin-secreting mesenchymal cells from adjacent joints deposit within adventitial layer of vessel walls during embryogenesis, and secrete mucin later in life ("developmental theory")
- Presentation
    - Intermittent claudication in otherwise young, healthy patient
- Risk factors
    - Male gender (5:1 ratio), average age of onset at 40 yo
- Management
    - Diagnosis
        - CT/MR angiogram (gold standard)
        - Conventional angiogram
            - Scimitar sign (focal, eccentric, smooth stenosis)

    - Hourglass deformity with circumferential cysts
  - Treatment
    - Surgical options
      - Percutaneous cyst aspiration (first line)
      - Open cyst resection
      - Popliteal artery resection with interposition graft
      - Endovascular repair not recommended due to prompt return of symptoms

DIABETIC FOOT ULCERS (DFU)

- Etiology
  - Repetitive trauma to feet leads to ulcer formation
    - Sensory neuropathy prevents sensation of pain and allows ulcer to develop
    - Motor neuropathy results in pedal deformities which predispose to ulceration
  - Ulcers can extend to deep tissue, become infected, and result in sepsis or osteomyelitis
- Presentation
  - Foot or ankle ulcers with or without underlying infection
- Classification (WIFI)
  - Wound
    - Grade 0: no ulcer, no gangrene
    - Grade 1: small ulcer, no gangrene
    - Grade 2: deep ulcer with limited toe gangrene
    - Grade 3: extensive ulcer or extensive gangrene
  - Ischemia
    - Graded based on TP or TcpO2
      - Toe pressure (TP) if ABI is compressible (ABI <1.3)

    - Transcutaneous oxygenation pressure (TcpO2) if incompressible
  - Grade 0: ≥60 mmHg
  - Grade 1: 40-59 mmHg
  - Grade 2: 30-39 mmHg
  - Grade 3: <30 mmHg
- Foot infection
  - Grade 0: no infection
  - Grade 1: mild infection (<2 cm cellulitis)
  - Grade 2: moderate infection (>2 cm cellulitis or purulence)
  - Grade 3: severe infection (sepsis)

- Risk factors
  - Sustained hyperglycemia with poorly controlled diabetes
  - Best predictor of ulcer development is previous ulcer
- Management
  - Diagnosis
    - Physical exam
      - Evaluate for purulence, probe to bone
    - Foot X-ray
      - Check for osteomyelitis
    - Lab tests
    - CBC (leukocytosis), BMP (hyperglycemia), ESR/CRP, wound cultures
    - CT angiogram
    - Conventional angiogram
    - Toe pressures
      - >40 mmHg indicates good healing potential (>60 mmHg in diabetics)
    - Laser perfusion tests
      - TcpO2 >40 indicates good healing potential
      - TcpO2 <30 indicates poor healing potential

- Treatment
  - Medical management
    - IV antibiotics (for infection)
  - Surgical options
    - Toe amputation
    - Transmetatarsal amputation
    - Formal amputation (BKA vs AKA)
    - Revascularization
      - ✓ Indicated for TcpO2 <40

Femoral Artery Aneurysm (FAA)

- Etiology
  - CFA diameter >150% normal
  - Most commonly due to atherosclerotic degeneration
- Presentation
  - Asymptomatic
  - Symptomatic
    - Lower extremity ischemia (chronic thrombosis)
    - Painful, pulsatile mass (local compression)
    - Can result in rupture or thromboembolization
- Classification
  - Type I FAA: involves CFA only
  - Type II FAA: involves CFA to PFA orifice
- Risk factors
  - Atherosclerosis (hypertension, hyperlipidemia, smoking, diabetes)
  - Male gender (20:1 ratio)
- Management
  - Diagnosis
    - Duplex ultrasound

      - Bilateral FAA in 70% of patients
    - CT/MR angiogram
    - Conventional angiogram
    - Abdominal ultrasound
      - AAA in 85% of patients
  - Treatment
    - Surgical options
      - Aneurysmectomy with interposition graft
      - Endovascular repair not recommended due to stent fracture at inguinal ligament
    - Indications for surgery
      - Symptomatic aneurysms, size >2.5 cm

INFECTED FEMORAL ARTERY PSEUDOANEURYSM

- Etiology
  - Infected pseudoaneurysm at femoral artery injection site
  - *Staphylococcus aureus* is most common organism
- Presentation
  - Pulsatile, tender groin mass with cellulitis and serosanguineous drainage
  - Femoral neuropathy (nerve compression)
  - Femoral vein thrombosis (local inflammation)
  - Can result in rupture, thromboembolization, septic shock
- Risk factors
  - IV drug abuse, arterial catheterization
- Management
  - Diagnosis
    - Duplex ultrasound
    - CT/MR angiogram
      - Differentiate PSA from abscess or hematoma

        - Conventional angiogram
    - Treatment
        - Medical management
            - IV antibiotics
        - Surgical options
            - Debridement and arterial ligation alone
            - Debridement and arterial ligation with revascularization
                - ✓ Obturator foramen bypass
                - ✓ Axillo-femoral bypass
                - ✓ Axillo-popliteal bypass

Popliteal Artery Aneurysm (PAA)

- Etiology
    - Popliteal artery diameter >150% normal
    - Most commonly due to atherosclerotic degeneration
- Presentation
    - Asymptomatic
    - Symptomatic
        - Acute limb ischemia (thrombosis)
        - Blue toe syndrome (digital embolization)
        - Tibial/peroneal neuropathy (nerve compression)
- Management
    - Diagnosis
        - Duplex ultrasound (bilateral)
            - 40% of PAA patients have bilateral PAA
        - CT/MR angiogram
        - Conventional angiogram
            - Useful for bypass planning

        - Need 2+ vessel runoff, 2 cm proximal/distal landing zones
      - Abdominal ultrasound
        - 50% of PAA patients have AAA
    - Treatment
      - Surgical options
        - Exclusion with femoro-popliteal bypass graft
          - ✓ Medial approach allows GSV harvesting, more familiarity
          - ✓ Posterior approach allows easier aneurysm decompression
        - Covered stent insertion (*Viabahn*®)
        - Catheter-directed TPA
          - ✓ Indicated for category I or IIa acute limb ischemia only
        - Amputation
          - ✓ Indicated for category III acute limb ischemia
      - Indications for surgery
        - Size >2.0 cm, symptomatic, intramural thrombus

ATHEROEMBOLISM

- Etiology
  - Distal embolization of atherosclerotic plaque debris to small arteries and arterioles
  - Embolization usually triggered by instrumentation or anticoagulation but can occur spontaneously
- Presentation

  - Blue toe syndrome: acute onset, painful cyanotic toes with scattered petechiae, livedo reticularis
  - Atheroembolic renal disease (AERD): renal failure, hypertension, eosinophilia
  - Internal iliac involvement can result in acute erectile dysfunction
  - Ascending aortic involvement can result in ischemic stroke
- Risk factors
  - Atherosclerosis (hypertension, hyperlipidemia, smoking, diabetes, male gender)
- Management
  - Diagnosis
    - CT/MR angiogram
    - Echocardiogram
      - Rule-out cardiac source
    - Hypercoagulable work-up
  - Treatment
    - Medical management
      - Aspirin, statin
      - Supportive care, avoid further instrumentation
      - Anticoagulation (controversial)
    - Surgical options
      - Treat embolic source
      - Pedal embolectomy via popliteal cutdown
      - Pedal artery bypass grafting
      - Catheter-directed TPA
        - ✓ Best used as an adjunct rather than primary therapy

Extremity Compartment Syndrome

- Etiology
    - Prolonged ischemia (>4-6 hrs) causes reperfusion injury to muscles
    - Results in muscle swelling within fascia, which can compress veins, arteries, or nerves
- Presentation
    - 6 Ps – pain, pallor, parasthesias, paralysis, poikilothermia, pulselessness
    - First sign of leg compartment syndrome is numbness in first webspace secondary to deep peroneal nerve compression in anterior compartment
- Management
    - Diagnosis
        - Physical exam
            - Tight compartments
            - Severe pain on passive motion
        - Compartment pressures
            - Compartment pressure >30 mmHg
            - Delta pressure <30 mmHg
            - Diastolic minus compartment pressures
    - Treatment
        - Four-compartment fasciotomy
    - Prevention
        - Prophylactic fasciotomy
            - Indicated for revascularization with ischemic time >4-6 hrs

Chapter 5

MESENTERIC REVIEW

OVERVIEW

- Acute Embolic Mesenteric Ischemia
- Acute Thrombotic Mesenteric Ischemia
- Non-occlusive Mesenteric Ischemia (NOMI)
- Mesenteric Venous Thrombosis
- Chronic Mesenteric Ischemia
- Median Arcuate Ligament Syndrome (MALS)
- Superior Mesenteric Artery (SMA) Syndrome
- Visceral Artery Aneurysms

ACUTE EMBOLIC MESENTERIC ISCHEMIA

- Etiology
    - Embolic occlusion of SMA due to oblique origin from aorta
        - 1/3 of acute occlusive mesenteric ischemia cases
    - Acute SMA occlusion results in ischemia of small bowel and colon

        - 15% lodge at SMA ostium
        - 50% lodge distal to middle colic and jejunal branches due to caliber change
            - Spares proximal jejunum and transverse colon as result of distribution
        - 35% lodge distally after fragmentation
    - 20% have synchronous emboli
- Presentation
    - Sudden-onset diffuse mid-abdominal pain "out of proportion" to examination, nausea/emesis, diarrhea
- Risk factors
    - Atrial fibrillation (75%), myocardial infarction, rheumatic heart disease, LV aneurysm, endocarditis
- Management
    - Diagnosis
        - CT angiogram
            - Evaluate for bowel ischemia, synchronous emboli
        - Mesenteric angiogram
            - Sharp cutoff at proximal healthy SMA with poor collaterals
    - Treatment
        - Medical management
            - Fluid resuscitation, antibiotics
            - Anticoagulation
        - Surgical options
            - Exploratory laparotomy
                - ✓ Possible bowel resection
                - ✓ Consider second-look operation
            - SMA embolectomy
            - SMA thrombolysis

Acute Thrombotic Mesenteric Ischemia

- Etiology
  - Acute on chronic thrombotic occlusion of SMA secondary to low flow or plaque rupture
    - 2/3 of acute occlusive mesenteric ischemia cases
- Presentation
  - Sudden-onset diffuse mid-abdominal pain "out of proportion" to examination, nausea/emesis, diarrhea
  - Often have history of chronic mesenteric ischemia (e.g., postprandial abdominal pain, food fear, weight loss)
- Risk factors
  - Atherosclerosis (hypertension, hyperlipidemia, smoking)
- Management
  - Diagnosis
    - CT angiogram
      - Evaluate for bowel ischemia
    - Mesenteric angiogram (gold standard)
      - Shaggy cutoff at diseased SMA with developed collaterals
      - GDA-PDA collaterals (celiac-SMA)
      - Arc of Riolan, marginal artery of Drummond (SMA-IMA)
      - Hemorrhoidal collaterals (IMA-hypogastric)
  - Treatment
    - Medical management
      - Fluid resuscitation, antibiotics
      - Anticoagulation
    - Surgical options
      - Exploratory laparotomy
        - ✓ Possible bowel resection
        - ✓ Consider second-look operation

- SMA endarterectomy with patch angioplasty
- Mesenteric bypass
  - ✓ Antegrade bypass from aorta
  - ✓ Retrograde bypass from CIA (usually right)
- SMA angioplasty/stenting
- SMA thrombolysis

Non-Occlusive Mesenteric Ischemia (NOMI)

- Etiology
  - o Vasoconstriction of SMA leads to intestinal hypoperfusion and ischemia
- Presentation
  - o Diffuse abdominal pain "out of proportion" to examination, nausea/emesis, diarrhea
  - o Symptoms can be unreliable in intubated and critically ill patients
- Risk factors
  - o Elderly, low volume (e.g., post-dialysis), pressor support, digitalis, cocaine
- Management
  - o Diagnosis
    - ▪ CT angiogram
    - ▪ Mesenteric angiogram (Siegelman criteria)
      - – Narrowing of SMA branch origins
      - – "String of sausages" sign – alternating dilation and narrowing
      - – Spasm of mesenteric arcades
      - – Impaired filling of intramural branches
  - o Treatment
    - ▪ Medical management

    - Treat underlying cause
    - Avoid pressors
  - Intra-arterial papaverine
    - 24 hrs via SMA catheterization
    - 60 mg/hr in NS (incompatible in LR)
    - Repeat arteriogram afterwards

Mesenteric Venous Thrombosis

- Etiology
  - Thrombosis of mesenteric veins (SMV, splenic vein, portal vein)
  - Hematologic causes include hypercoagulable states, oral contraceptives
  - Nonhematologic causes include pancreatitis, diverticulitis, cirrhosis, trauma, low-flow states
- Presentation
  - Acute symptoms
    - Sudden-onset diffuse mid-abdominal pain "out of proportion" to examination
  - Subacute symptoms
    - Gradually worsening abdominal pain (diffuse, colicky)
    - Most common presentation
  - Chronic symptoms
    - Asymptomatic, found incidentally on imaging
- Risk factors
  - Hypercoagulable states, oral contraceptives, pancreatitis, cirrhosis
- Management
  - Diagnosis
    - CT with delayed venous phase

        - Venous filling defects in SMV/PV
        - Bowel edema, mesenteric stranding, ascites
      - Mesenteric venous duplex
      - Rule-out hypercoagulable disorders
  - Treatment
      - Medical management
        - Anticoagulation
        - Bowel rest
      - Surgical options
        - Catheter-directed TPA
          - ✓ Can be indirect (into SMA), transjugular, or transhepatic
          - ✓ Rarely used, indicated for acute SMV/PV thrombosis

Chronic Mesenteric Ischemia

- Etiology
  - Stenosis of mesenteric vessels causes decreased intestinal perfusion
    - Atherosclerosis is most common etiology (90-95%)
    - Other etiologies include fibromuscular dysplasia, vasculitis, dissection, drug-induced, radiation
  - Requires stenosis of two (of three) mesenteric vessels
- Presentation
  - Chronic diffuse mid-abdominal pain ("intestinal angina")
  - Food fear, weight loss, malnutrition, nausea/emesis
- Risk factors
  - Female gender (80%)
  - Atherosclerosis (hypertension, hyperlipidemia, smoking)
- Management

- Diagnosis
  - Mesenteric duplex (fasting)
    - 50% stenosis
      - ✓ Celiac EDV >55 cm/sec or retrograde common hepatic flow
      - ✓ SMA EDV >45 cm/sec
    - 70-99% stenosis
      - ✓ Celiac PSV >200 cm/sec
      - ✓ SMA PSV >275 cm/sec
  - CT/MR angiogram
  - Mesenteric angiogram (gold standard)
    - Multiplanar views
- Treatment
  - Surgical options
    - SMA angioplasty/stenting (1st line)
  - Balloon-expandable covered stent (*iCast*®, *VBX*®)
      - ✓ Primary patency 50% at 3 years
    - "Trapdoor" mesenteric endarterectomy
    - Mesenteric bypass (gold standard)
      - ✓ Antegrade bypass from aorta
        - ❖ Single-vessel or multi-vessel bypass
        - ❖ Preferred due to short graft, no kinking, direct inline flow
        - ❖ No difference in antegrade vs retrograde patency
      - ✓ Retrograde bypass from CIA (usually right)
        - ❖ Useful for avoiding aortic cross-clamping
    - Retrograde open mesenteric stenting (ROMS)
  - Indications for surgery
    - Symptomatic stenosis >70%

Median Arcuate Ligament Syndrome (MALS, Dunbar Syndrome)

- Etiology
  - Median arcuate ligament of diaphragm causes extrinsic compression of celiac axis
  - Low-lying median arcuate ligament and high origin of celiac artery predispose to compression
  - Controversial diagnosis
- Presentation
  - Postprandial abdominal pain, food fear, abdominal bruits
- Risk factors
  - Young age, female gender
- Management
  - Diagnosis
    - Rule-out alternative diagnoses
    - Mesenteric duplex (1st line)
      - Celiac PSV >200, EDV <55 cm/sec
    - CT/MR angiogram
    - Mesenteric angiogram (gold standard)
      - Celiac narrowing on superior aspect just distal to origin
      - Maximal compression with full expiration
  - Treatment
    - Surgical options
      - Open median arcuate ligament release
      - Laparoscopic median arcuate ligament release
      - Celiac artery angioplasty/stenting

Superior Mesenteric Artery (SMA) Syndrome (Wilkie Syndrome)

- Etiology
  - Rapid weight loss causes SMA to compress 3rd segment of duodenum
- Presentation
  - Proximal SBO (early satiety, frequent bilious emesis)
- Risk factors
  - Female gender, low BMI, young age (10-40 yo)
- Management
  - Diagnosis
    - CT angiogram
      - Narrow aortomesenteric angle (<25°)
    - Barium swallow
      - Abrupt cutoff at D3 segment
  - Treatment
    - Medical management
      - Weight gain
      - May need feeding tube past obstruction
    - Surgical options
      - Laparoscopic duodenojejunostomy
      - Open duodenojejunostomy
    - Indications for surgery
      - Failure of medical management

Visceral Artery Aneurysms

- Etiology
  - Visceral artery diameter >150% normal

- Multiple etiologies depending on affected artery
  - Celiac - medial degeneration (MCC), post-stenotic dilation
  - Hepatic - trauma (MCC intrahepatic), medial degeneration (MCC extrahepatic)
  - Splenic - increased splenic blood flow during pregnancy (MCC), medial fibrodysplasia, portal hypertension, chronic pancreatitis, trauma
  - GDA/PDA - high-flow from celiac stenosis (MCC true aneurysms), pancreatitis (MCC pseudoaneurysms)
  - SMA - medial degeneration (MCC), mycotic aneurysms, trauma
  - IMA - high-flow IMA secondary to celiac and SMA occlusive disease (MCC)
  - Jejunal/ileal/colic - mycotic aneurysms (MCC), arteriopathy - polyarteritis nodosa, Behcet disease, segmental mediolytic arteritis

- Presentation
  - Asymptomatic (majority)
  - Symptomatic
    - Celiac - nonspecific abdominal pain, mass effect (early satiety, jaundice), rupture (hemoperitoneum)
    - Hepatic - mass effect (jaundice), rupture into peritoneal cavity (hemoperitoneum) or biliary tree (hemobilia)
    - Splenic - rupture into lesser sac (back pain) followed by peritoneal cavity ("double rupture phenomenon")
    - GDA/PDA - abdominal pain, rupture into peritoneal cavity (hemoperitoneum) or GI tract (massive GI bleed)
    - SMA - acute expansion (epigastric/back pain), dissection (mesenteric ischemia), or rupture (hemoperitoneum)

        - IMA - symptomatic with pulsatile abdominal mass, rupture
        - Jejunal/ileal/colic - abdominal pain (majority), rupture
- Diagnosis
    - CT/MR angiogram
    - Conventional angiogram
- Treatment
    - Surgical options
        - Celiac artery aneurysms
            - Aneurysmectomy with/without reconstruction
                - ✓ Aorto-celiac bypass
                - ✓ Aorto-hepatic artery bypass
            - Endovascular repair not recommended due to early branching, compression at median arcuate ligament
        - Extrahepatic artery aneurysms
            - Aneurysmectomy with/without reconstruction
                - ✓ Reconstruction indicated for poor GDA collateral flow
            - Covered stent placement
        - Intrahepatic artery aneurysms
            - Angioembolization
            - Liver resection
            - Liver transplantation
        - Splenic artery aneurysms
            - Aneurysmectomy (proximal)
            - Splenectomy (distal)
            - Covered stent placement
            - Angioembolization
        - GDA/PDA aneurysms
            - Angioembolization
            - Aneurysmectomy/aneurysm ligation
        - SMA aneurysms

      - Aneurysmectomy with reconstruction
        - ✓ Aorto-SMA bypass
        - ✓ Aorto-SMA reimplantation
      - Covered stent placement
    - IMA aneurysms
      - Aneurysmectomy with/without reconstruction
    - Jejunal/ileal/colic aneurysms
      - Coil embolization (first line)
      - Aneurysmectomy/aneurysm ligation
  - Indications for surgery
    - Celiac - symptomatic, size >2 cm, all pseudoaneurysms
    - Hepatic - symptomatic, size >2 cm, growth >5 mm/yr, positive blood cultures, vasculitis
    - Splenic - symptomatic, size >3 cm (not 2 cm), growth >5 mm/yr, all pseudoaneurysms, women of childbearing age
    - GDA/PDA - all aneurysms
    - SMA - all aneurysms
    - IMA - symptomatic, size >2 cm
    - Jejunal/ileal - symptomatic, size >2 cm, all pseudo-aneurysms
    - Colic - all aneurysms

Chapter 6

RENOVASCULAR REVIEW

OVERVIEW

- Renal Artery Stenosis (RAS)
- Renal Artery Dissection
- Atheroembolic Renal Disease (AERD)
- Renal Artery Aneurysm
- Renal Vein Thrombosis
- Renal Arteriovenous Malformation (AVM)

RENAL ARTERY STENOSIS (RAS)

- Etiology
    - Renal artery stenosis secondary to multiple etiologies
        - Atherosclerosis (80%)
            - Involves renal ostia from aortic spillover (2/3) or focal plaque (1/3)
        - Fibromuscular dysplasia (15%)

        - Involves distal main renal artery and branches
        - Bilateral in 55% of patients
      - Dissection, trauma, developmental hypoplasia, Takayasu arteritis (5%)
        - Renovascular hypertension is most common presenting sign of TA
- Presentation
  - Asymptomatic
  - Symptomatic with renovascular hypertension, ischemic nephropathy, or recurrent heart failure (flash pulmonary edema)
    - Renovascular hypertension (5% of hypertension cases)
      - Poor renal perfusion results in release of renin
      - Angiotensinogen -[renin]→ AT I -[ACE]→ AT II → aldosterone release
      - AT II causes vasoconstriction, hypertension
      - Aldosterone causes sodium retention, volume expansion
    - Ischemic nephropathy
      - Poor renal perfusion results in progressive renal insufficiency
- Risk factors
  - Atherosclerosis - male gender, advanced age, smoking, diabetes, hyperlipidemia
  - Fibromuscular dysplasia - female gender, young age
- Management
  - Diagnosis
    - Duplex ultrasound
      - Normal: PSV <180 cm/s, RAR <3.5
      - <60% stenosis: PSV >180 cm/s, RAR <3.5, post-stenotic turbulence

        - >60% stenosis: PSV >180 cm/s, RAR >3.5, post-stenotic turbulence
    - CT/MR angiogram
        - Risk of contrast-induced nephropathy (CT)
        - Risk of nephrogenic systemic fibrosis (MR, GFR <30)
    - Conventional angiogram
        - Pressure gradient >10-15 mmHg
- Treatment
    - Medical management
        - Aspirin, smoking cessation, exercise, healthy diet
        - Treat hypertension (<140/90), diabetes (A1c <7%), hyperlipidemia (LDL <100 or <70 for diabetics)
        - ACE inhibitors are first-line for renovascular hypertension
    - Surgical options
        - Renal bypass graft
            - ✓ Aorto-renal bypass
                - ❖ GSV or PTFE (6 mm) ideal for adults
                - ❖ Hypogastric artery ideal for kids
            - ✓ Ilio-renal bypass
            - ✓ Spleno-renal bypass (left)
            - ✓ Hepato-renal bypass (right)
        - Trans-aortic renal endarterectomy
        - Renal angioplasty (for FMD)
            - ✓ Rescue stenting reserved for suboptimal results or flow-limiting dissection
        - Renal angioplasty/stenting (for atherosclerosis)
        - Renal auto-transplantation
    - Indications for surgery
        - Symptomatic stenosis (>60%) with one of the following

        - ✓ Accelerated or refractory hypertension
        - ✓ Rapidly deteriorating renal function (esp. in absence of proteinuria)
        - ✓ Recurrent flash pulmonary edema or heart failure
      - – Open repair preferred for small diameter (<6 mm), long stenosis (>15 mm), early bifurcation, concomitant aortic surgery, Takayasu arteritis, or failure of endovascular intervention
      - – Endovascular repair preferred for poor surgical candidates, hostile abdomen, short life expectancy (<5 yrs)
    - ▪ Indicators of renal recovery after revascularization
      - – Renal resistive index (RRI) >0.8 is poor prognostic factor
      - – Atrophic kidney or size difference >1 cm is poor prognostic factor
- Studies
  - o ASTRAL trial: revascularization has no benefit over medical management (renal dysfunction)
  - o CORAL trial: revascularization has no benefit over medical management (death, stroke, MI, hospitalization, renal dysfunction)
  - o RAOOD trial: open repair has higher primary patency (88% vs 68%) and cumulative patency (90% vs 80%, 4 yrs) vs endovascular repair

RENAL ARTERY DISSECTION

- Etiology
  - o Intimal tear within renal artery

- Primary dissection associated with underlying atherosclerosis or FMD
- Secondary dissection results from blunt trauma or vascular procedures

- Presentation
  - Asymptomatic
  - Symptomatic with renovascular hypertension, ischemic nephropathy, flank/back pain, hematuria
- Management
  - Diagnosis
    - CT/MR angiogram
    - Conventional angiogram
      - Most common method of detecting iatrogenic dissection
  - Treatment
    - Medical management
      - Observation
      - Treatment of underlying hypertension
    - Surgical options
      - Renal artery bypass
      - Renal auto-transplantation
      - Nephrectomy
        - ✓ Indicated for worsening clinical status without any options for arterial reconstruction
        - ✓ Avoid early nephrectomy when possible due to potential for spontaneous improvement
      - Renal artery stenting
        - ✓ Ideal for focal dissections confined to main renal artery
        - ✓ Branch involvement precludes endovascular stenting
    - Indications for surgery

- Controversial
- Low chance of success for revascularization if >4 hrs warm ischemia time

ATHEROEMBOLIC RENAL DISEASE (AERD)

- Etiology
  - Cholesterol plaque embolization to renal arteries
  - Primary atheroemboli result from spontaneous plaque dislodgement
  - Secondary atheroemboli result from anticoagulation or vascular procedures
- Presentation
  - Acute AERD
    - Renal failure <1 week of inciting event
    - Associated with gastrointestinal and cutaneous emboli
  - Subacute AERD
    - Renal failure weeks-months after inciting event
    - Average onset is 5 weeks
  - Chronic AERD
    - Asymptomatic
    - Symptomatic with insidious renal failure not specifically tied to inciting event
    - Difficult to diagnose clinically due to delayed onset
- Risk factors
  - Atherosclerosis (hypertension, hyperlipidemia, smoking, diabetes, male gender)
- Management
  - Diagnosis
    - Physical exam

- Cutaneous findings after invasive procedure are pathognomonic
- Lab studies
  - Urinalysis (proteinuria, hematuria)
  - CBC (eosinophilia)
- Kidney biopsy
- Skin biopsy
- Fundoscopy
  - Cholesterol crystals (Hollenhorst plaques)

- Treatment
  - Medical management
    - Avoid inciting events
      - ✓ Anticoagulation (controversial), vascular procedures
    - Aspirin, smoking cessation, exercise, healthy diet
    - Treat hypertension (<140/90), diabetes (A1c <7%), hyperlipidemia (LDL <100 or <70 for diabetics)

RENAL ARTERY ANEURYSM

- Etiology
  - Renal artery diameter >150% normal
  - Majority are saccular and tend to occur at bifurcations
- Presentation
  - Asymptomatic
  - Symptomatic with renovascular hypertension or ischemic nephropathy
    - Occurs with aneurysmal thrombus or embolization
    - Rupture can result in retroperitoneal hemorrhage or hemoperitoneum
- Management

- Diagnosis
  - CT/MR angiogram
  - Conventional angiogram
- Treatment
  - Surgical options
  - Aneurysmectomy with primary closure
    - Aneurysmectomy with reconstruction
      - ✓ Reimplantation for branch artery aneurysms
      - ✓ Aorto-renal bypass for main artery aneurysms
    - Covered stent placement
      - ✓ Can be difficult with branch aneurysms
    - Renal auto-transplantation
  - Indications for surgery
    - Symptomatic, size >3 cm, women of childbearing age

Renal Vein Thrombosis

- Etiology
  - Thrombosis of renal vein
  - Left renal vein more commonly affected than right renal vein (3:1 ratio)
- Presentation
  - Acute renal vein thrombosis
    - Symptomatic with acute-onset flank pain, hematuria, renal failure
    - Kidney rupture can lead to fatal retroperitoneal hemorrhage
  - Chronic renal vein thrombosis
    - Asymptomatic
    - Renovascular hypertension

    - Ischemic nephropathy
- Risk factors
  - Neonatal/pediatric population
    - Severe dehydration (sepsis, diarrhea, toxemia)
  - Adult population
    - Nephrotic syndrome (urinary loss of AT III)
    - Renal cell carcinoma, extrinsic compression, hypercoagulability, suprarenal IVC filters
- Management
  - Diagnosis
    - Duplex ultrasound
      - Bidirectional renal artery flow (due to venous obstruction)
    - CT/MR venogram
    - Conventional venogram
  - Treatment
    - Medical management
      - Anticoagulation
    - Surgical options
      - Catheter-directed TPA
        - ✓ Both renal artery and vein
      - Open thrombectomy
        - ✓ Indicated for failure of thrombolysis
      - Nephrectomy
        - ✓ Indicated for acute capsular rupture
      - Suprarenal IVC filter
        - ✓ Indicated for failure or contraindication to anticoagulation
    - Indications for surgery
      - Impaired renal function, bilateral thrombosis, solitary kidney with thrombosis, transplanted kidney with thrombosis, or significant IVC involvement

Renal Arteriovenous Malformation (AVM)

- Etiology
    - Abnormal connection between renal artery and vein
    - Congenital AV malformations involve multiple feeding arteries
    - Acquired AV fistulas have a solidary feeding artery
        - Iatrogenic causes include biopsy (most common), percutaneous nephrostomy, lithotripsy
        - Other causes include trauma (blunt/penetrating), neoplasm, or aneurysms
- Presentation
    - Asymptomatic
    - Symptomatic with hematuria (most common), hypertension, high-output heart failure
- Management
    - Diagnosis
        - Duplex ultrasound
            - Turbulent flow, elevated PSV and EDV
        - CT/MR angiogram
        - Conventional angiogram
    - Treatment
        - Observation
            - First-line for small, asymptomatic fistulas
        - Surgical options
            - Angioembolization
            - Covered stent insertion
            - Partial nephrectomy
            - Nephrectomy
        - Indications for surgery

- Symptoms (gross hematuria, high-output heart failure, worsening renovascular hypertension, worsening ischemic nephropathy)

Chapter 7

VENOUS REVIEW

OVERVIEW

- Superficial Venous Thrombosis (SVT)
- Deep Venous Thrombosis (DVT)
- May-thurner Syndrome
- Pulmonary Embolism (PE)
- Paradoxical Embolism
- Chronic Venous Insufficiency (CVI)
- Superior Vena Cava (SVC) Syndrome
- Vena Cava Tumors
- Nutcracker Syndrome
- Pelvic Congestion Syndrome

Superficial Venous Thrombosis (SVT)

- Etiology
    - Thrombosis of superficial vein
- Presentation
    - Palpable venous cord
    - Suppurative thrombophlebitis: superinfected thrombosis causes erythema, fluctuance, fever
    - Mondor disease: superficial thrombosis of anterior chest wall/breast
    - Trousseau phenomenon: pancreatic adenocarcinoma produces mucins, resulting in migratory SVTs
- Risk factors
    - Smoking, obesity, pregnancy, OCPs, malignancy, trauma, family history
- Management
    - Diagnosis
        - Physical exam
        - Duplex ultrasound
    - Treatment
        - Medical management
            - NSAIDs, warm compresses
            - Fondaparinux
                - ✓ 2.5 mg subcutaneous x 45 days (CALISTO trial)
                - ✓ Indicated for high-risk patients - affected vein segment >5 cm or within <5 cm from saphenofemoral/saphenopopliteal junction
        - Surgical options
            - Thrombophlebectomy
        - Indications for surgery
            - Suppurative thrombophlebitis

DEEP VENOUS THROMBOSIS (DVT)

- Etiology
  - Thrombosis of deep vein
- Presentation
  - Unilateral extremity pain, swelling
    - 10% have concomitant PE, 1% have phlegmasia
  - Phlegmasia alba dolens (PAD)
    - Severe pain/swelling with pallor
    - Massive DVT impairs venous outflow
  - Phlegmasia cerulea dolens (PCD)
    - Severe pain/swelling with cyanosis
    - Massive DVT impairs venous outflow resulting in tissue edema, which impairs arterial perfusion
- Risk factors
  - Smoking, obesity, pregnancy, OCPs, malignancy, trauma, family history
- Management
  - Diagnosis
    - Duplex ultrasound
      - Noncompressible lumen, enlarged vein, hypoechoic thrombus
    - CT/MR venogram
    - Conventional venogram
  - Treatment
    - Medical management
      - Observation (distal to knee)
      - Anticoagulation (proximal to knee)
        - ✓ DOAC (most patients)
        - ✓ Warfarin (APLS patients)
        - ✓ LMWH (pregnant or cancer patients)
    - Surgical options

- IVC filter
  - ✓ Indicated for failure or contraindication to anticoagulation
  - ✓ Filter removal failure rate is highest with duration >7 months
- Catheter-directed TPA
  - ✓ 0-1% risk of intracerebral hemorrhage
- Percutaneous mechanical thrombectomy
- Open thrombectomy
  - ✓ Only used if CDT not available
- Indications for surgery
  - ✓ PAD/PCD

- ▪ Prevention
  - Mechanical prophylaxis
  - Subcutaneous heparin/LMWH

- Studies
  - o PREPIC trial: IVC filter decreases risk of PE, increases risk of DVT, no change in mortality (at 8 yr follow-up)

MAY-THURNER SYNDROME

- Etiology
  - o R iliac artery compresses L iliac vein, resulting in L iliofemoral DVT
  - o 25-30% of population have asymptomatic L iliac vein compression
- Presentation
  - o L lower extremity pain, swelling
- Management
  - o Diagnosis
    - ▪ Duplex ultrasound

        - CT/MR venogram
        - Conventional venogram
    - Treatment
        - Medical management
            - Anticoagulation
        - Surgical options
            - Catheter-directed TPA
        - Percutaneous mechanical thrombectomy
            - ✓ Indicated for severe acute thrombosis
        - L iliac vein angioplasty/stent
            - ✓ Best measured using IVUS with 50% reduction in vein size
            - ✓ Oversize venous stent by 10-15%

PULMONARY EMBOLISM (PE)

- Etiology
    - Embolization of above-knee DVT vs low-flow state
- Presentation
    - Sinus tachycardia, pleuritic chest pain, hemoptysis, cardiogenic shock
- Risk factors
    - Smoking, obesity, pregnancy, OCPs, malignancy, trauma, family history
- Classification
    - Submassive PE: severe RV dysfunction or myocardial necrosis
    - Massive PE: hemodynamic instability
- Management
    - Diagnosis
        - CTPA

        - Gold standard
    - V/Q scan
        - If no underlying lung disease
    - ABG
        - ↑pH, ↓pO2, ↓pCO2
    - Echocardiogram
        - Evaluate for right heart strain
    - EKG
        - Sinus tachycardia is most common finding
        - S1Q3T3 is less common but pathognomonic
    - D-dimer
        - Rule-out PE if negative
- Treatment
    - Medical management
        - Anticoagulation
    - Surgical options
        - IVC filter
            - ✓ Indicated for failure or contraindication to anticoagulation
        - If submassive →
            - ✓ Catheter-directed TPA
            - ✓ Catheter-directed mechanical thrombectomy
        - If massive →
            - ✓ Systemic TPA
            - ✓ Pulmonary embolectomy (Trendelenburg procedure)
            - ✓ ECMO cannulation
    - Indications for surgery
        - Submassive or massive PE

Paradoxical Embolism

- Etiology
  - Venous embolism passes through right-to-left shunt and lodges in arterial bed
  - Most common cause is patent foramen ovale
  - Other causes include VSD, PDA, pulmonary AV fistula
- Presentation
  - Consider with simultaneous VTE and acute arterial ischemia
  - Cryptogenic stroke with PFO is not diagnostic of paradoxical embolism
- Management
  - Diagnosis
    - Echocardiogram
      - Bubble study can detect right-to-left shunt
      - Impending paradoxical embolus (clot in both right and left atria) is diagnostic
    - Transcranial Doppler
      - Bubble study can detect right-to-left shunt but can't localize location of shunt
  - Treatment
    - Medical management
      - Anticoagulation
    - Surgical options
      - IVC filter
        - ✓ Indicated for lower extremity source with contraindication to anticoagulation
      - Treat arterial embolism
      - PFO closure
        - ✓ Indicated for PFO with paradoxical embolism
        - ✓ Not indicated for PFO with cryptogenic stroke

- ✓ No difference in time to recurrent stroke or death

Chronic Venous Insufficiency (CVI)

- Etiology
  - Chronic venous hypertension
- Presentation
  - Lower extremity edema, varicose veins, skin changes, venous ulcers
- Risk factors
  - Prior DVT (post-thrombotic), obesity, pregnancy, smoking, female sex
  - Personal and family history of DVT are risk factors for progression (Edinburgh Vein Study)
- Classification (CEAP)
  - Clinical signs
    - C0: no clinical signs
    - C1: telangiectasias, reticular veins
    - C2: varicose veins
    - C3: edema
    - C4: skin changes (hyperpigmentation, LDS, eczema)
    - C5: healed venous ulceration
    - C6: active venous ulceration
  - Etiology
    - EC: congenital
    - EP: primary
    - ES: secondary (post-thrombotic)
  - Anatomy
    - AS: superficial veins
    - AD: deep veins

        - AP: perforating veins
    - Pathophysiology
        - PR: reflux
        - PO: obstruction
        - PRO: reflux and obstruction
- Management
    - Diagnosis
        - Venous duplex ultrasound
            - Standing or steep reverse Trendelenburg with outward leg rotation
            - Valsalva maneuver used to elicit venous reflux
            - Pathologic reflux is >1 sec for femoral and popliteal veins; >0.5 sec for deep femoral, saphenous, tibial veins; >0.5 sec and diameter >3.5 mm for perforator veins
    - Treatment
        - Medical management
            - Compression therapy
                - ✓ First-line for C1-C5
            - Unna boot
                - ✓ Calamine/zinc gauze with ACE wrap
                - ✓ First-line for C6 (active ulcers)
            - Pentoxifylline, sulodexide, flavonoids
        - Surgical options
            - GSV ablation
                - ✓ Prevents ulcer recurrence
                - ✓ Contraindicated with acute or recurrent DVTs, critical limb ischemia, infection
            - Stab phlebectomy
            - Sclerotherapy
            - Ulcer debridement

- ✓ Indicated for venous ulcers with devitalized tissue
- ▪ Indications for surgery
  - – Failure of medical management (>3 months)

Superior Vena Cava (SVC) Syndrome

- Etiology
  - o Intraluminal obstruction or extrinsic compression of SVC
  - o Multiple causes including lung cancer (most common cause), indwelling catheters, mediastinal fibrosis
- Presentation
  - o Unilateral or bilateral upper extremity and head/neck edema, worse with lying down
  - o Severe cases can cause dyspnea, dysphagia, hoarseness, upper airway compromise
- Management
  - o Diagnosis
    - ▪ CT/MR venogram
      - – Conventional venogram
  - o Treatment
    - ▪ Medical management
      - – Upright positioning, diuresis
      - – IV steroids
      - – Radiation therapy (malignancy)
    - ▪ Surgical options
      - – SVC angioplasty/stenting (first line)
      - – Open SVC angioplasty
    - ▪ Indications for surgery
      - – Failure of medical management

VENA CAVA TUMORS

- Etiology
  - Primary or secondary tumor of the vena cava
    - Most common primary tumor is leiomyosarcoma
    - Most common secondary tumor is renal cell carcinoma
  - Can lead to IVC or SVC obstruction
  - Majority of cases are metastatic at time of diagnosis
- Presentation
  - IVC obstruction leads to lower extremity edema, varicose veins, abdominal wall varices
  - SVC obstruction leads to dyspnea, SVC syndrome, cardiac dysfunction
- Management
  - Diagnosis
    - CT/MR venogram
    - Transesophageal echocardiogram
      - Evaluate for cardiac tumor thrombus
    - CT chest
      - Metastatic work-up
  - Treatment
    - Surgical options
      - Radical resection
        - ✓ Surgical exposure
          - ❖ SVC - median sternotomy
          - ❖ Retrohepatic cava - right 8th interspace thoracoabdominal incision
          - ❖ IVC - midline laparotomy
        - ✓ Radical resection
        - ✓ Caval reconstruction
          - ❖ Femoral vein, spiral GSV, PTFE grafts

            - ❖ Not necessary in chronic occlusion with good collateral flow
        - – SVC/IVC angioplasty/stenting
            - ✓ Indicated for unresectable tumors
    - ▪ Indications for surgery
        - – Primary vena cava leiomyosarcoma, non-metastatic, with good cardiopulmonary function

NUTCRACKER SYNDROME

- Etiology
    - o Left renal vein compression
        - ▪ Anterior nutcracker syndrome: compression of left renal vein between aorta and SMA
        - ▪ Posterior nutcracker syndrome: compression of retroaortic left renal vein between aorta and vertebral column
    - o Rare causes of left renal vein compression include lymphadenopathy, malignancy, retroperitoneal fibrosis
- Presentation
    - o Asymptomatic (nutcracker phenomenon)
    - o Symptomatic (nutcracker syndrome)
        - ▪ Men can present with chronic pelvic/flank pain, hematuria, left-sided varicocele
        - ▪ Woman can present with chronic pelvic/flank pain, hematuria, vulvar varices, dyspareunia, dysuria
- Risk factors
    - o Female gender, low BMI (lack of retroperitoneal fat)
- Management
    - o Diagnosis
        - ▪ Duplex ultrasound

- Elevated left renal vein PSV
- CT/MR venogram
  - Left renal vein compression
  - Decreased aortomesenteric angle
- Conventional venogram
  - Gold standard
  - Reno-caval gradient >3 mmHg
- Treatment
  - Observation
    - Indicated for asymptomatic or mildly symptomatic patients
    - Many patients will resolve symptoms on their own
  - Surgical options
    - Left renal vein transposition
      - ✓ Gold standard
    - Left reno-caval bypass with GSV
    - Left renal vein stenting
      - ✓ Oversize by 20%
      - ✓ Extend stent into IVC
  - Indications for surgery
    - Severe or persistent symptoms

Pelvic Congestion Syndrome

- Etiology
  - Chronic venous hypertension of the pelvic veins
  - Two main hypotheses
    - Ovarian vein valvular dysfunction
    - Internal iliac venous hypertension
- Presentation
  - Chronic pelvic pain (noncyclic, lasting >6 months)

    - May also have symptoms of lower extremity chronic venous insufficiency
- Risk factors
    - Female gender, multigravida, retroverted uterus, PCOS
- Management
    - Diagnosis
        - Gynecologic examination
        - Venous duplex ultrasound
        - CT/MR venogram
        - Conventional venogram
            - Ovarian vein reflux
            - Venous flow crossing midline
            - Pelvic varicose veins
    - Treatment
        - Surgical options
            - Ovarian vein coil embolization
            - Laparoscopic ovarian vein ligation
            - Open ovarian vein ligation
        - Indications for surgery
            - Symptomatic abnormal venous reflux

Chapter 8

LYMPHATIC REVIEW

OVERVIEW

- Groin lymphocele
- Lymphocutaneous fistula (LCF)
- Lymphedema

GROIN LYMPHOCELE

- Etiology
  - Cystic collection of lymphatic fluid from disrupted lymphatic channel
- Presentation
  - Painless, pulseless soft mass in groin
  - Painful, erythematous mass indicates infected lymphocele or abscess
- Risk factors
  - Operative technique, inguinal lymphadenopathy, redo groin dissection, extensive groin dissection

    - Incidence is 1% for initial operations, 8% for redo operations
- Management
    - Diagnosis
        - Duplex ultrasound
        - CT scan (noncontrast)
        - Needle aspiration
            - Useful for diagnostic uncertainty only
            - Low protein content (0.5-2.0 g/dL), clear aspirate, lymphocytes
    - Treatment
        - Observation
        - Needle aspiration (if large)
        - Treat extremity edema
            - Compression stockings, leg elevation
    - Prevention
        - Meticulous surgical dissection, ligation of visible lymphatic channels, multi-layered closure
        - Transverse groin incision (vs vertical incision) is debatable

LYMPHOCUTANEOUS FISTULA (LCF)

- Etiology
    - Uncontained and draining lymphatic fluid from a recent groin wound
- Presentation
    - Persistent wound drainage or high JP drain output
    - Can exceed >500 ml per day
    - High risk of developing wound and graft infection
- Risk factors

- Operative technique, inguinal lymphadenopathy, redo groin dissection, extensive groin dissection
- Incidence is 1% for initial operations, 8% for redo operations

- Management
  - Diagnosis
    - Clinical judgment
  - Treatment
    - Medical management
      - Prophylactic antibiotics (*Ancef*)
      - Wound VAC placement
        - ✓ Alternative for low-output, uncomplicated fistulas
      - Treat extremity edema
        - ✓ Compression stockings, leg elevation
    - Surgical options
      - Early wound exploration
        - ✓ Obtain bacterial culture at time of exploration
        - ✓ Isosulfan blue injection can help identify lymphatics
        - ✓ Excise fibrous pseudocapsule
        - ✓ Local rotational muscle flap to close dead space
    - Indications for surgery
      - Uncontrolled or high-output fistulas
  - Prevention
    - Meticulous surgical dissection, ligation of visible lymphatic channels, multiple layered closure
    - Transverse groin incision (vs vertical incision) is debatable

LYMPHEDEMA

- Etiology
  - Pathologic accumulation of interstitial lymphatic fluid
  - Develops when fluid accumulation exceeds the lymphatic transport capacity
  - Chronic lymphedema results in interstitial fibrosis and fatty tissue deposition
- Presentation
  - Grade 0: subclinical/latent stage; no edema despite impaired lymphatic transport
  - Grade I: reversible stage; painless, soft, pitting edema that resolves with overnight elevation
  - Grade II: irreversible stage; thickened skin, non-pitting edema that doesn't resolve with overnight elevation
  - Grade III: lymphostatic elephantiasis; elephant skin (hardened skin with papillomata), extreme swelling
- Classification
  - Primary lymphedema
    - Develops without underlying cause
    - Congenital lymphedema: primary lymphedema onset <1 yo
    - Lymphedema praecox: primary lymphedema onset 1-35 yo
    - Lymphedema tarda: primary lymphedema onset >35 yo
  - Secondary lymphedema
    - Develops as a result of malignancy (nodal disease), radiation, lymphadenectomy, filariasis, etc.
- Management
  - Diagnosis
    - Physical exam

- Stemmer sign: inability to pinch thickened skin fold at base of second toe
- CT/MRI
  - Rule-out other causes of edema
- Lymphoscintigraphy
  - Dermal backflow, absent or delayed transport of the tracer, crossover filling with retrograde backflow, absent/delayed visualization of lymph nodes
- Lymphangiogram
  - Rarely performed except in setting of surgical planning

- Treatment
  - Medical management
    - Treat underlying cause
    - Complex decongestive therapy (CDT, first-line)
      - ✓ Leg elevation
      - ✓ Compression stockings
        - ❖ Class 3 garments (40-50 mmHg)
      - ✓ Skin care
        - ❖ Wash with soap/water, lubricate with emollient cream
      - ✓ Exercise program
      - ✓ Lymphatic massage
  - Surgical options
    - Excisional procedures
      - ✓ Tissue resection
      - ✓ Liposuction
      - ✓ Charles procedure
        - ❖ Radical resection with skin grafting

- Lymphatic reconstruction
    - ✓ Lymphovenous anastomosis
- Indications for surgery
    - Failure of medical management (>6 months)

Chapter 9

VASCULAR TRAUMA REVIEW

OVERVIEW

- Cerebrovascular Injury
- Blunt Thoracic Aortic Injury (BTAI)
- Thoracic Vascular Injury
- Abdominal Vascular Injury
- Retroperitoneal Hematoma (RPH)
- Extremity Vascular Injury
- Blunt Popliteal Artery Injury
- Extremity Compartment Syndrome
- Cold-related Injury

CEREBROVASCULAR INJURY

- Etiology
  - Penetrating or blunt injury to carotid or vertebral arteries

- Can be iatrogenic injury (e.g., chiropractors, central lines, spine surgery)
- Presentation
  - Hard signs: active bleeding, expanding or pulsatile hematoma, fixed neurologic deficit, palpable thrill, bruits, hemodynamic instability
  - Soft signs: non-expanding hematoma, proximity to major artery, cranial nerve injury, worrisome mechanism
- Classification (Denver)
  - Penetrating cerebrovascular injury
  - Blunt cerebrovascular injury (BCVI)
    - Grade I: intimal irregularity; or dissection/hematoma with <25% stenosis
    - Grade II: intimal flap or thrombus; or dissection/hematoma with >25% stenosis
    - Grade III: pseudoaneurysm
    - Grade IV: occlusion
    - Grade V: transection
- Management
    - Diagnosis
    - CT angiogram
    - Conventional angiogram
    - Surgical exploration
      - Indicated for hard signs and/or hemodynamic instability
  - Treatment
    - Medical management
      - Trauma resuscitation
      - Aspirin vs anticoagulation
        - ✓ Indicated for BCVI grades I-II
        - ✓ No great comparison studies
    - Surgical options

      - Neck exploration
        - ✓ Avoid passing Fogarty in distal carotid artery
      - Endovascular repair
        - ✓ Indicated for BCVI grades III-IV
  - Screening
    - CT angiogram
    - Denver screening criteria
      - Indicated for blunt injuries with GCS <8, C-spine fractures, Le Fort II/III, skull base fractures, DAI, hanging injury, seatbelt sign above clavicle, neurologic deficits, or infarcts on head CT

BLUNT THORACIC AORTIC INJURY (BTAI)

- Etiology
  - Rapid deceleration causes aorta to tear at ligamentum arteriosum distal to left subclavian artery
- Presentation
  - >80% mortality at scene of injury
  - Chest/back pain, interscapular murmur, pulse pressure deficit, hemorrhagic shock
  - Associated with fractures in thoracic spine, sternum, ribs, scapula
- Classification (SVS)
  - Grade I: intimal tear
  - Grade II: intramural hematoma
  - Grade III: pseudoaneurysm
  - Grade IV: rupture

- Management
    - Diagnosis
        - Chest X-ray
            - Widened mediastinum (>6 cm), obscured aortic knob, apical cap, depressed left mainstem bronchus, deviated NG tube, left hemothorax
            - 95% negative predictive value
        - CT angiogram
            - 100% sensitivity
        - Conventional angiogram
        - Transesophageal echocardiogram
    - Treatment
        - Medical management
            - Impulse control
            - Esmolol gtt, nicardipine gtt
        - Surgical options
            - TEVAR (first-line)
                - ✓ Can be delayed for other life-threatening injuries if stable
                - ✓ Consider left carotid-subclavian bypass for zone 2 injuries
            - Open aortic repair
                - ✓ Thoracic aorta - left anterolateral thoracotomy (4th interspace)
                - ✓ Abdominal aorta - exploratory laparotomy, left medial visceral rotation (supramesocolic), division of ligament of Treitz (inframesocolic)
        - Indications for surgery
        - Grade III (urgent) or IV (emergent)

THORACIC VASCULAR INJURY

- Etiology
  - Penetrating or blunt injury to aorta, innominate, subclavian, common carotid arteries
- Presentation
  - Hemorrhagic shock, cardiac tamponade, mortality
  - Commonly associated injuries - lung, brachial plexus, major veins
- Management
  - Diagnosis
    - CT angiogram
    - Conventional angiogram
    - Surgical exploration
  - Treatment
    - Initial management
      - Trauma resuscitation
    - Surgical options
      - Open exposure
        - ✓ Aortic arch injury - median sternotomy
        - ✓ Innominate injury - median sternotomy
        - ✓ Common carotid injury - median sternotomy
        - ✓ Right subclavian injury - median sternotomy (proximal), supraclavicular incision (distal)
        - ✓ Left subclavian injury - anterolateral thoracotomy (proximal), supraclavicular incision (distal)
        - ✓ Axillary artery - infraclavicular incision
        - ✓ Descending aortic injury - posterolateral thoracotomy
      - Primary repair
      - Repair with interposition graft

- Ligation
- Endovascular stenting
  - ✓ Disadvantages include inability to evacuate hematoma (can cause nerve compression), inability to address concomitant venous injuries, distal embolization of thrombus, stent compression/fracture

ABDOMINAL VASCULAR INJURY

- Etiology
  - o Penetrating or blunt injury to aorta, visceral branches, vena cava, portal venous system
- Presentation
  - o Hemoperitoneum, hemorrhagic shock, mortality
- Management
  - o Diagnosis
    - ▪ FAST exam
      - Screening test for blunt trauma
    - ▪ CT angiogram
    - ▪ Conventional angiogram
    - ▪ Exploratory laparotomy
  - o Treatment
    - ▪ Initial management
      - Trauma resuscitation
    - ▪ Surgical options
      - Open exposure
        - ✓ IVC - right medial visceral rotation
        - ✓ Retrohepatic IVC - total vascular isolation
          - ❖ Aortic cross-clamp below diaphragmatic hiatus, Pringle maneuver for portal triad,

suprarenal IVC control with umbilical tape, suprahepatic IVC control
- ✓ Celiac artery - lesser sac through gastrohepatic ligament
- ✓ Hepatic artery - right medial visceral rotation, Kocher maneuver
- ✓ Portal vein - left medial visceral rotation
- ✓ SMA - left medial visceral rotation (proximal), trans-mesenteric (distal)
- ✓ Renal artery - right medial visceral rotation (right), left medial visceral rotation (left)
    - ❖ Consider nephrectomy with life-threatening hemorrhage
- – Primary repair
- – Repair with interposition graft
- – Ligation
- – Endovascular stenting
    - ✓ Disadvantages include inability to evacuate hematoma (can cause nerve compression), inability to address concomitant venous injuries, distal embolization of thrombus, stent compression/fracture

RETROPERITONEAL HEMATOMA (RPH)

- Etiology
    - o Penetrating or blunt injury to retroperitoneal structures
- Presentation
    - o Central, perinephric, or pelvic hematoma
    - o Missed with FAST and DPL exams
- Classification (anatomic)

  - Zone 1: injury to pancreas, duodenum, or major abdominal vessels
  - Zone 2: injury to colon or genitourinary tract
  - Zone 3: injury to pelvic vessels, usually secondary to pelvic fracture
- Management
  - Diagnosis
    - CT angiogram
    - Exploratory laparotomy
  - Treatment
    - Initial management
      - Trauma resuscitation
    - Surgical options
      - Exploratory laparotomy
      - Angioembolization
    - Indications for exploration
      - All penetrating injuries
      - Blunt injuries in zone 1 (all) or zone 2 (expanding/pulsatile)

EXTREMITY VASCULAR INJURY

- Etiology
  - Penetrating or blunt injury to extremity arteries
- Presentation
  - Soft signs: prior hemorrhage, non-pulsatile hematoma, ABI <0.9
  - Hard signs: active hemorrhage, pulse deficit, expanding or pulsatile hematoma, distal ischemia, bruits/thrill
- Management
  - Diagnosis

    - Ankle-brachial index
      - Screening test
      - ABI <0.9 is abnormal
    - CT angiogram
      - Indicated for soft signs
    - Conventional angiogram
    - Surgical exploration
      - Indicated for hard signs
  - **Treatment**
    - Initial management
      - Trauma resuscitation
      - Direct manual pressure
      - Tourniquet use
        - ✓ Lowest pressure possible, time <2 hrs
      - Reduce fracture if present
    - Surgical options
      - Open exploration
      - Primary repair
        - ✓ Indicated for defects <2 cm without tension
      - Repair with interposition graft
        - ✓ Indicated defects >2 cm or significant tension
        - ✓ Vein graft preferred due to contamination
      - Temporary shunting
        - ✓ Indicated for hemodynamically unstable patients
      - Ligation
        - ✓ Acceptable if collateral flow is present
      - Endovascular covered stenting
        - ✓ Alternative option for patients who are hemodynamically stable, larger vessel size (>6 mm), minimal thrombosis, minimal soft tissue defects, difficult anatomic exposure (e.g., axillary/subclavian injury)

    - Extremity fasciotomy
        - ✓ Indicated for ischemic time >4-6 hrs
    - Primary amputation
        - ✓ Indicated for non-salvageable extremity

Blunt Popliteal Artery Injury

- Etiology
    - Injury to popliteal artery secondary to knee fracture or dislocation
    - Can result in dissection, thrombosis, embolization, transection
- Presentation
    - Abnormal pedal pulses in setting of ipsilateral knee injuries
    - 6 Ps – pain, pallor, parasthesias, paralysis, poikilothermia, pulselessness
- Management
    - Diagnosis
        - Physical exam
            - Check for distal pulses
        - ABI
            - <0.9 is abnormal
            - Reduce fracture if present
        - CT angiogram
            - Gold standard
        - Conventional angiogram
    - Treatment
        - Initial management
            - Trauma resuscitation
        - Surgical options
            - Open exploration

- ✓ Primary repair
  - ❖ Indicated for defects <2 cm without tension
- ✓ Repair with interposition graft
  - ❖ Indicated defects >2 cm or significant tension
  - ❖ Vein graft preferred due to contamination
- ✓ Temporary shunting
  - ❖ Indicated for hemodynamically unstable patients
  - ❖ Useful for temporary revascularization during fracture fixation

- – Endovascular covered stenting
- – Extremity fasciotomy
  - ✓ Indicated for ischemic time >4-6 hrs
- – Primary amputation
  - ✓ Indicated for non-salvageable extremity

EXTREMITY COMPARTMENT SYNDROME

- Etiology
  - o Elevated soft tissue pressures within an inelastic compartment
  - o Multiple etiologies
    - ▪ IV fluid infiltration
    - ▪ Ischemia-reperfusion injury
    - ▪ Prolonged ischemia (>4-6 hrs) causes reperfusion injury to muscles
    - ▪ Results in muscle swelling within fascia, which can compress veins, arteries, or nerves

        - Circumferential burn eschar
        - Iatrogenic (dressings, casts, splints)
- Presentation
    - 6 Ps – pain, pallor, parasthesias, paralysis, poikilothermia, pulselessness
    - First sign of leg compartment syndrome is numbness in first webspace secondary to deep peroneal nerve compression in anterior compartment
- Management
    - Diagnosis
        - Physical exam
            - Tight compartments
            - Severe pain on passive motion
            - Unreliable in sedated patients
        - Lab tests
            - CK levels indicate muscle necrosis
        - Compartment pressures
            - Compartment pressure >30 mmHg
            - Delta pressure <30 mmHg
                - Diastolic minus compartment pressures
        - Duplex ultrasound
            - Normal venous size/function rules-out compartment syndrome
    - Treatment
            - Extremity fasciotomy
    - Prevention
            - Prophylactic fasciotomy
            - Indicated for revascularization with ischemic time >4-6 hrs

COLD-RELATED INJURY

- Etiology
  - Localized cold injury produced at freezing temperatures
  - Vasoconstriction results in progressive vascular thrombosis and local ischemia
  - Freezing of tissue cause ice crystal formation resulting in mechanical trauma
- Presentation
  - Superficial frostbite: pallor, parasthesias, blistering, reactive hyperemia with rewarming
  - Deep frostbite: insensate, painful, progresses to full-thickness necrosis with rewarming
- Risk factors
  - Armed conflict (e.g., trench warfare), outdoor sports
- Classification
  - Non-freezing injuries
    - Chilblain
    - Immersion foot
    - Trench foot
  - Freezing injuries (frostbite)
    - 1st degree: hyperemia, edema
    - 2nd degree: hyperemia, clear vesicles
    - 3rd degree: partial-thickness skin necrosis, hemorrhagic vesicles
    - 4th degree: full-thickness skin necrosis
- Management
  - Diagnosis
    - Physical exam
  - Treatment
    - Initial management
      - Immerse in 104-108°C agitated water bath

  - Continue 15 minutes beyond thawing (digital flush)
  - Local wound care
    - ✓ Debride clear blisters
    - ✓ Keep hemorrhagic blisters intact
    - ✓ Topical aloe vera
- Surgical options
  - Intra-arterial TPA
    - ✓ Indicated for severe frostbite within 24 hrs of injury
    - ✓ No benefit after 24 hrs post-injury
  - Debridement
    - ✓ Indicated for devitalized tissue
    - ✓ Allow necrotic tissue to demarcate for several weeks prior to debridement
  - Amputation
    - ✓ Indicated for extensive deep tissue necrosis

Chapter 10

DIALYSIS ACCESS REVIEW

OVERVIEW

- Chronic Kidney Disease (CKD)
- Access Failure
- Access Bleeding
- Access-related Hand Ischemia (Steal Syndrome)
- Ischemic Monomelic Neuropathy (IMN)

CHRONIC KIDNEY DISEASE (CKD)

- Etiology
  - Progressive loss of kidney function over months to years
- Presentation
  - Asymptomatic
  - Symptomatic with electrolyte or acid-base imbalances, fluid overload, hypertension, uremia
- Classification
  - CKD stage 1: GFR $\geq$90

- CKD stage 2: GFR 60-89
- CKD stage 3: GFR 30-59
- CKD stage 4: GFR 15-29
- CKD stage 5 (ESRD): GFR <15 or dialysis

- Risk factors
  - Diabetes, hypertension, heart disease, family history of kidney failure, acute kidney injury
- Management
  - Pre-access evaluation
    - Ask about dominant handedness, prior central venous access, upper extremity trauma
    - Physical exam
      - Allen test
      - Check for intact palmar arch
      - Evaluate for central venous stenosis - unilateral arm swelling, prominent veins
    - Arterial duplex
    - Vein mapping
      - Requires 3 mm veins, 2 mm arteries
  - Access options
    - Upper extremity AV fistula
      - Distal > proximal
        - ✓ Radiocephalic > brachiocephalic > brachio-basilic
        - ✓ Basilic vein transposition can be single stage if >4 mm
      - Non-dominant arm > dominant arm
      - Patency rates
        - ✓ AV fistula primary patency 55% at two years
        - ✓ AV graft primary patency 40% at two years
      - Rule of 6's
        - ✓ Defines when fistula access is ready for use

      - ✓ 6 mm diameter
      - ✓ Flow >600 ml/min
      - ✓ 6 mm from surface of skin
      - ✓ 4-6 weeks post-op
  - Upper extremity AV graft
    - Indicated if no fistula options available
    - Tapered (4-7 mm) or non-tapered (6 mm) PTFE options
    - No difference in steal, patency, or complication rates
    - Early access grafts can be accessed within 24 hrs
    - Hybrid catheter/graft (HeRO graft)
      - ✓ Indicated for central venous stenosis
      - ✓ Graft made of 6 mm PTFE connected to 19 Fr venous outflow catheter
  - Dialysis catheter
    - Indicated for urgent/emergent hemodialysis
    - Non-tunneled dialysis catheters
    - Tunneled dialysis catheters
      - ✓ Can be used up to 12 months
  - Lower extremity AV fistula
    - Indicated for central venous occlusion
    - Femoral vein transposition
    - Saphenous vein transposition
    - Rule-out PAD prior to placement
  - Peritoneal dialysis catheter
    - Requires patient education and good compliance
- Indications for access surgery
  - NKF KDOQI guidelines
    - CKD stage 4 (CrCl <25 ml/min) or 5
  - AV fistula 6 months prior to anticipated dialysis
  - AV graft 3-6 weeks prior to anticipated dialysis

Access Failure

- Etiology
  - Poor arterial inflow or venous stenosis
- Presentation
  - Low flow rates during hemodialysis
  - Prolonged bleeding from puncture site indicates central venous stenosis
- Risk factors
  - Prior central venous access, upper extremity trauma
- Management
  - Diagnosis
    - Physical exam
    - Graft duplex
    - Fistulogram
  - Treatment
    - If graft stenosis →
      - Balloon angioplasty
        - ✓ 2-3 minute insufflation
      - Vein patch angioplasty
      - Interposition vein graft
    - If graft thrombosis →
      - Catheter-directed TPA
      - Suction thrombectomy
      - Open thrombectomy

Access Bleeding

- Etiology
  - Repeated access puncture results in degeneration and possible pseudoaneurysm formation

- Presentation
  - Spontaneous bleeding from fistula/graft site
  - Hemorrhagic shock with delayed presentation
- Management
  - Diagnosis
    - Physical exam
      - Hold pressure on wound
    - Fistulogram
      - Evaluate for central venous stenosis
  - Treatment
    - Surgical options
      - Revision of fistula/graft
      - Treat any underlying venous stenosis
    - Indications for surgery
      - Active bleeding, ulceration, significant skin thinning

ACCESS-RELATED HAND ISCHEMIA (STEAL SYNDROME)

- Etiology
  - Inadequate blood flow distal to fistula/graft results in ischemic symptoms
- Presentation
  - Asymptomatic
  - Symptomatic with cramping hand pain and coolness
    - Compression of fistula/graft alleviates symptoms
- Classification
  - Grade 0: asymptomatic
  - Grade 1: mild ischemia, asymptomatic with cool extremity
  - Grade 2: moderate ischemia, symptomatic during dialysis
  - Grade 3: severe ischemia, symptomatic at rest, tissue loss
- Management

- Diagnosis
  - Physical exam
  - Graft duplex ultrasound
    - Arterial flow reversal distal to access site
  - Digital plethysmography
- Treatment
  - Surgical options
    - Distal revascularization with interval ligation (DRIL)
    - Revision using distal inflow (RUDI)
    - Fistula banding
    - Fistula/graft takedown
  - Indications for surgery
    - Grades 2 and 3

Ischemic Monomelic Neuropathy (IMN)

- Etiology
  - Steal syndrome involving distal nerves
- Presentation
  - Severe, intractable neuropathic hand pain and forearm muscle weakness
  - Hand remains warm with intact pulses
  - Occurs several hours after fistula/graft creation
- Risk factors
  - Diabetes
- Management
  - Diagnosis
    - Physical exam
  - Treatment
    - Emergent fistula/graft takedown

Chapter 11

Miscellaneous Review

Overview

- Access-related Hematoma
- Access-related Pseudoaneurysm (PSA)
- Access-related Retroperitoneal Hematoma (RPH)
- Access-related Vasovagal Syndrome
- Access-related Arteriovenous (AV) Fistula
- Access-related Limb Ischemia
- Heparin-induced Thrombocytopenia (HIT)
- Warfarin-induced Skin Necrosis
- Congenital Hypercoagulable Disorders
- Marfan Syndrome
- Vascular Ehlers-Danlos Syndrome (VEDS)
- Loeys-Dietz Syndrome

ACCESS-RELATED HEMATOMA

- Etiology
  - Incomplete hemostasis with contained blood clot after arterial catheterization
- Presentation
  - Pain, mass at access site, overlying ecchymosis
  - Brachial sheath hematoma may present with symptoms of median nerve palsy (numbness/parasthesias in fingers 1-3) *without* any external signs of underlying hematoma
- Risk factors
  - Hypertension (most common), large diameter cannulation, female gender (smaller arteries), anticoagulation, profunda cannulation, obesity (can't hold adequate pressure), lack of ultrasound guidance
- Management
  - Diagnosis
    - Physical exam
    - Duplex ultrasound
    - CT angiogram
  - Treatment
    - Medical management
      - Observation
      - Manual pressure
    - Surgical options
      - Hematoma evaluation
    - Indications for surgery
      - Skin necrosis, nerve compression, hemodynamic instability
      - *Emergent* evacuation indicated for brachial sheath hematoma

ACCESS-RELATED PSEUDOANEURYSM (PSA)

- Etiology
  - Rupture of arterial wall with blood contained in a fibrous capsule after arterial catheterization
- Presentation
  - Pain, pulsatile mass at access site, overlying ecchymosis
  - Hematoma can also be pulsatile with transmission of underlying pulse
- Risk factors
  - Hypertension (most common), large diameter cannulation, female gender (smaller arteries), anticoagulation, profunda cannulation, obesity (can't hold adequate pressure), lack of ultrasound guidance
- Management
  - Diagnosis
    - Physical exam
    - Duplex ultrasound
    - CT angiogram
  - Treatment
    - Medical management
      - Observation
      - Ultrasound-guided compression therapy
      - Ultrasound-guided thrombin injection
        - ✓ May not be feasible with small PSA or short neck
    - Surgical options
      - Open pseudoaneurysm repair
    - Indications for surgery
      - Failure of thrombin injection, short/wide neck not amenable to thrombin injection, rapidly expanding, active bleeding, skin necrosis, or nerve compression

Access-Related Retroperitoneal Hematoma (RPH)

- Etiology
    - Incomplete hemostasis into retroperitoneum after arterial catheterization
- Presentation
    - Abdominal/back pain, femoral neuralgia
    - Unexplained hypotension or hemoglobin drop may indicate an undetected RPH after femoral access
- Risk factors
    - Punctures above the inguinal ligament, lack of ultrasound guidance
- Management
    - Diagnosis
        - Physical exam
        - CT angiogram
    - Treatment
        - Surgical options
            - Covered stent placement
            - Open surgical repair
        - Indications for surgery
            - Nerve compression, hemodynamic instability, active extravasation

Access-Related Vasovagal Syndrome

- Etiology
    - Exaggerated parasympathetic response to pain
    - Most common systemic complication after arterial access

- Presentation
  - Hypotension, bradycardia, nausea, pallor, diaphoresis
- Management
  - Diagnosis
    - Clinical judgment
    - Rule-out hemorrhage
  - Treatment
    - Medical management
      - IV fluids
      - Atropine (rarely needed)

Access-Related Arteriovenous (AV) Fistula

- Etiology
  - Direct communication between artery and vein
- Presentation
  - Asymptomatic
  - Holosystolic/diastolic bruits over catheter site
- Management
  - Diagnosis
    - Physical exam
    - Duplex ultrasound
  - Treatment
    - Medical management
      - Observation
      - Most AV fistulas resolve on their own
      - Follow with serial duplex ultrasound
    - Surgical options
      - Open surgical repair
    - Indications for surgery

- Limb ischemia, venous insufficiency, congestive heart failure

ACCESS-RELATED LIMB ISCHEMIA

- Etiology
    - Thrombosis, embolization, or dissection following arterial catheterization
- Presentation
    - Change in pulse examination following arterial access procedure
    - Acute limb ischemia with prolonged flow-limiting lesions
- Risk factors
    - Technical difficulties with closure devices
- Management
    - Diagnosis
        - Physical examination
            - Change in pulse exam
        - Duplex ultrasound
        - Pulse volume recordings
    - Treatment
        - Medical management
            - Anticoagulation
        - Surgical options
            - Open thromboembolectomy
            - Endovascular stenting (for dissections)

HEPARIN-INDUCED THROMBOCYTOPENIA (HIT)

- Etiology
  - Type 1 HIT: heparin directly binds platelets
  - Type 2 HIT: anti-PF4 antibodies cause platelet activation and thrombosis
- Presentation
  - Type 1 HIT
    - Mild thrombocytopenia within 4 days of initiation
  - Type 2 HIT
    - Moderate to severe thrombocytopenia from 4-10 days of initiation
    - 50% present with acute thromboembolic event
    - Also referred to as heparin-induced thrombocytopenia with thrombosis (HITT)
- Management
  - Diagnosis
    - 4T score (pretest screening tool)
      - Thrombocytopenia with >50% platelet drop
      - Timing within 5-10 days
      - Thrombosis or skin necrosis
      - other causes ruled out
    - Anti-PF4 IgG ELISA
      - Screening test
    - Serotonin-release assay (SRA)
      - Confirmation test
  - Treatment
    - If type I →
      - Observation
    - If type II →

- Discontinue heparin until diagnostic tests are negative
- Avoid platelet transfusion unless symptomatic
- Alternative anticoagulation if thromboses are present
  - ✓ Bivalirudin (renal metabolism)
  - ✓ Argatroban (hepatic metabolism)
  - ✓ Fondaparinux (prophylaxis)

WARFARIN-INDUCED SKIN NECROSIS

- Etiology
  - o Warfarin initiation results in a temporary hypercoagulable state due to protein C/S inhibition
  - o Almost all cases of warfarin-induced skin necrosis result from not appropriately bridging warfarin with alternative anticoagulant (e.g., unfractionated heparin, low molecular weight heparin)
- Presentation
  - o Necrotic skin lesion occurring within 24-72 hrs after initiation of warfarin
- Risk factors
  - o Protein C deficiency, HITT, DIC, APLS
- Management
  - o Diagnosis
    - ▪ Physical exam
    - ▪ Lab tests
      - – Prolonged PT/PTT
      - – Elevated D-dimer
      - – Thrombocytopenia

- Treatment
  - Supportive care
- Prevention
  - Bridge warfarin with UFH or LMWH until therapeutic (INR 2.0)

Congenital Hypercoagulable Disorders

- Etiology
  - Factor V Leiden
    - Most common hypercoagulable disorder
    - Mutation in factor V causes activated protein C resistance
    - Recurrent thrombosis noted in homozygous but *not* heterozygous mutations
  - Prothrombin G21210A
    - Second most common hypercoagulable disorder
    - Mutation in prothrombin causes inappropriate activation of fibrinogen
    - Not at risk for recurrent thrombosis
  - Antithrombin III deficiency
    - Deficient AT III (<70%) causes inability to inhibit clotting cascade
    - Increased risk of heparin-resistant thrombosis
  - Antiphospholipid syndrome
    - Antiphospholipid antibodies cause endothelial dysfunction with production of TXA2 and tissue factor
  - Homocysteinemia
    - Elevated serum homocysteine levels
  - Protein C deficiency

        - Mutation in PC causes inability to inhibit clotting cascade
        - Increased risk of warfarin-induced skin necrosis
    - Protein S deficiency
        - Mutation in PS causes inability to inhibit clotting cascade
        - PS acts as cofactor for PC
        - Increased risk of warfarin-induced skin necrosis
- Presentation
    - Venous and arterial thromboses
- Management
    - Diagnosis
        - Hypercoagulability panel
            - AT III activity/antigen, prothrombin G21210 assay, anti-cardiolipin antibody, homocysteine levels, factor VIII assay, activated PC resistance, PC activity/antigen, PS antigen, dilute Russell viper venom test
            - Indicated for young age (<40 yrs), idiopathic thrombosis, recurrent thrombosis, family history, and unusual locations
    - Treatment
        - Lifelong anticoagulation
            - Indicated for all congenital hypercoagulable disorders (except for prothrombin G21210 and heterozygous factor V Leiden)

Marfan Syndrome

- Etiology
    - *ΔFBN1* (fibrillin) on chromosome 15

  - Autosomal dominant (75%), de novo mutation (25%)
    - 1 in 5,000 individuals
- Presentation
  - Vascular features
    - Aortic root and thoracic aortic aneurysms/dissections
  - Non-vascular features
    - Tall/thin phenotype
    - Pectus carinatum/excavatum
    - Ectopia lentis (dislocated lenses)
    - Spontaneous pneumothorax
    - Mitral valve prolapse
- Management
  - Diagnosis
    - Ghent criteria
      - Aortic root dilation, ectopia lentis, family history, genetic tests
    - Genetic testing
  - Treatment
    - Medical management
      - Refer to multidisciplinary care team
      - Avoid burst-type exertional activities
      - Maintain resting HR <70, exercise HR <100
      - Minimize vascular interventions
    - Surgical principles
      - Open/hybrid repair > endovascular repair
      - Avoid vascular closure devices
    - Indications for surgery
      - Aortic root dilation >5 cm, thoracic aorta >5.5 cm

VASCULAR EHLERS-DANLOS SYNDROME (VEDS)

- Etiology
  - *ΔCOL3A1* (collagen type III)
  - Autosomal dominant
    - 1 in 50,000 individuals
- Presentation
  - Vascular features
    - Abdominal aortic aneurysms (no aortic root involvement)
    - Peripheral and visceral aneurysms
  - Non-vascular features
    - Thin, translucent skin
    - Spontaneous pneumothorax
    - Spontaneous bowel perforation
    - Spontaneous uterine rupture
- Management
  - Diagnosis
    - Genetic testing
  - Treatment
    - Medical management
      - Refer to multidisciplinary care team
      - Avoid burst-type exertional activities
      - Maintain resting HR <70, exercise HR <100
      - Minimize vascular interventions
    - Surgical principles
      - Open/hybrid repair > endovascular repair
      - Avoid vascular closure devices

LOEYS-DIETZ SYNDROME

- Etiology
  - *ΔTGFB1/TGFB2* (transforming growth factors)
  - Autosomal dominant (25%), de novo mutation (75%)
- Presentation
  - Vascular features
    - Aortic root and thoracic aortic aneurysms/dissections
    - Peripheral and visceral arterial aneurysms
  - Non-vascular features
    - Thin, translucent skin
    - Craniofacial dysmorphism - bifid uvula, cleft palate, hypertelorism
- Management
  - Diagnosis
    - Genetic testing
  - Treatment
    - Medical management
      - Refer to multidisciplinary care team
      - Avoid burst-type exertional activities
      - Maintain resting HR <70, exercise HR <100
      - Minimize vascular interventions
    - Surgical principles
      - Open/hybrid repair > endovascular repair
      - Avoid vascular closure devices

REFERENCES

Moore WS. *Moore's Vascular and Endovascular Surgery*. Elsevier; 2019.

Rasmussen TE, Clouse WD, Tonnessen BH. *Handbook of patient care in vascular diseases*. Philadelphia: Wolters Kluwer; 2019.

Sidawy AN, Perler BA, Rutherford RB. *Rutherford's vascular surgery and endovascular therapy*. Philadelphia, PA: Elsevier; 2019.

Stanley JC. *Current therapy in vascular and endovascular surgery*. Elsevier; 2014.

AUTHOR'S CONTACT INFORMATION

Young Kim, MD
Massachusetts General Hospital,
Boston, MA, US
ykim73@mgh.harvard.edu

INDEX

A

B

C

D

E

F

G

H

I

U

V

W